# RESERVATIONS
## *for*
# NINE

### A DOCTOR'S FAMILY
### CONFRONTS CANCER

## GEORGE BEAUREGARD
### FOREWORD BY CRAIG MELVIN

*Reservations for Nine*

Copyright © 2025 by George Beauregard. All rights reserved.

No part of this book may be used or reproduced in any manner whatsoever without written permission, except in the case of brief quotations embodied in critical articles and reviews. For more information, e-mail all inquiries to info@manhattanbookgroup.com.

Published by:

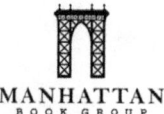

Manhattan Book Group
447 Broadway 2nd Floor, #354, New York, NY 10013
(212) 634-7677
www.manhattanbookgroup.com

Printed in the United States of America
ISBN-13: 978-1-965340-34-9

# CONTENTS

| | | |
|---|---|---|
| 1: | "All We Have Is Today" | 1 |
| 2: | The Marine | 13 |
| 3: | Misbehaving Cells | 23 |
| 4: | Opening Acts | 29 |
| 5: | The Doctor | 45 |
| 6: | Role Reversal | 55 |
| 7: | Before and After | 79 |
| 8: | "I Will Never Give Up" | 87 |
| 9: | Chemo Days | 109 |
| 10: | Reservations for Nine | 125 |
| 11: | Team Panda Power | 129 |
| 12: | Looking for a Breakthrough | 137 |
| 13: | Brothers | 149 |
| 14: | Glimmers of Hope | 157 |
| 15: | The Advocate | 165 |
| 16: | Rock Bottom | 171 |
| 17: | "He's Here!" | 175 |
| 18: | A Last Cape Vacation | 187 |
| 19: | Homecoming | 191 |
| 20: | Taps | 201 |
| 21: | Giving | 209 |
| 22: | Frontiers of Hope | 213 |
| 23: | Two Suitcases | 227 |
| 24: | Afterword | 237 |
| 25: | Acknowledgments | 245 |
| 26: | Bibliography | 247 |

| | |
|---|---|
| Dedications | 253 |
| Testimonial | 255 |
| Praise for Reservations for Nine | 257 |

# INVICTUS

Out of the night that covers me,
  Black as the Pit from pole to pole,
I thank whatever gods may be
  For my uncompromised soul.

In the fell clutch of circumstance
  I have not winced nor cried aloud.
Under the bludgeonings of chance
  My head is bloody, but unbowed.

Beyond this place of wrath and tears
  Looms but the Horror of the shade,
And yet the menace of the years
  Finds, and shall find, me unafraid.

It matters not how strait the gate,
  How charged with punishments the scroll,
I am the master of my fate:
  I am the captain of my soul.

—William Ernest Henry. 1849–1903

For my cherished grandsons, Noah and Colin:
May your lives be enriched by the indomitable
spirit that lived within your father. It will remain
forever beside you.

# "RESERVATION FOR NINE"— FOREWORD

## By Craig Melvin

I remember Patrick well. When traveling through life's darkest and deepest valleys, I've always been convinced God periodically sends rays of light to help us feel our way through to continue the journey. Patrick Beauregard was light personified. When he came to NBC's 'The TODAY Show' in March of 2020 to talk about his three-year battle with colorectal cancer, it took all the strength I could muster to hold it together during our interview. Here sat a handsome 29-year-old Marine veteran who'd been diagnosed with the same disease my brother was battling at the same time. On our couch in the studio, Patrick's beautifully beaming wife sat next to him looking on with pride. Their lives had been a whirlwind ever since they'd gotten married because he was diagnosed just four weeks after their wedding. As we listened to them share their love and cancer journey, you couldn't even tell Amanda was already four months pregnant with their first child. I fought back tears and swallowed hard thinking about how difficult all of this must be for her as a caregiver and an expecting new mom. Balancing worries while juggling doctor's visits for her and shuttling him to and from chemotherapy. While I marveled at their strength that morning, I also thought about my sister-in-law Angela. Her children were older, 9 and 7 at the time, but she had a demanding job and was traveling with Lawrence nearly every two weeks to MD Anderson in Texas for his treatment and meetings with doctors. Besides being diagnosed with a crushing disease in the prime of their lives, Patrick and Lawrence had something else in common. They had both become advocates and ambassadors for a cause.

We started doing more stories and segments on the show when Lawrence was diagnosed in 2017 about the alarming rise in cases among young people. We also showcased new treatments, research findings, and highlighted survivors who'd endured multiple surgeries, radiation, and chemo. We've shown what caregiving looks like up close and explained to our viewers how cancer doesn't just affect the patient, but all those who love him or her. We joined forces with a non-profit committed to finding a cure, the Colorectal Cancer Alliance. Eventually I joined their board as an unpaid member. Lawrence gave speeches. I did too. We criss crossed the country while he still could to talk about the importance of screenings and learning your family history. We were on a mission that's become a crusade to destigmatize conversations about colons, rectums, and blood in your stool. It helped give him a sense of purpose especially when it became apparent he wasn't going to live long enough to see his son and daughter grow up. Since his death in 2020 at age 43, my family and I along with the alliance and 'The TODAY Show' have stepped up our efforts to raise awareness. We use the show even more to encourage people to get screened, and my wife and I started a golf tournament when Lawrence died to raise awareness and money. In three years, we've raised $3.3 million for the Colorectal Cancer Alliance to fund research, pay for screenings, and support caregivers. We've used our pain for a purpose.

Patrick was an ally in the fight too. During his appearance on the show, he said "I tell people all the time and do everything I can to raise awareness and tell people to be an advocate." He added, "I am blessed that I am still here." After 40 rounds of chemo, the guy was grateful to be alive. After 20 years of interviewing people, you can get a decent sense of someone's spirt in just a few minutes. His was indomitable. I'd only known him a few minutes, but

I cried a little too when I heard he died just six months later. My brother, Lawrence Meadows, died three months after Patrick.

On our journey terribly unfair and inexplicable things happen—sickness, death, and grief. There's nothing we can do about that. All we can control is how we respond. 'Reservations for Nine' is a perfect response. The pages that follow chronicle Patrick's truly inspiring story and delves into the current state of cancer treatment. It reveals his family's hope then heartbreak while also exploring some of the causes behind the alarming rise in early onset cases of colorectal cancer. It's a love letter to Patrick and all of us who have seen up close how this dreadful disease robs children of their dads and it's a tribute to the tribes forced to carry on burdened by grief and sadness.

"In a situation like this, your mind can either liberate you or essentially incarcerate you…and you choose what to make of it."

—*Patrick Beauregard, appearing as a guest on the* Today Show, *March 10, 2020*

# 1

# "All We Have Is Today"

THE HANDSOME COUPLE stood before an arbor draped with flowers at the end of a pier jutting into Newport Harbor. It was the lovely summer evening of August 31, 2019, at the Bohlin, a tented venue at the Newport Yachting Center in Newport, Rhode Island, with the temperature in the low eighties and a gentle breeze coming off the shimmering Atlantic. More than 200 people were gathered to observe the ceremony. My oldest son, Daniel George Beauregard, was marrying Melissa Burtis Hart, his longtime girlfriend. As the couple exchanged vows, boats glided by in the water. People on board took notice and let out whoops and cheers.

Patrick Beauregard, my second son, officiated at the ceremony. At six feet, two inches, he stood a bit taller than his brother. Patrick has striking features, dark hair and straight polished teeth in a memorable smile. His hazel eyes signify a calm, yet penetrating intensity. Throughout the ceremony, he largely stuck to the script, but added occasional humorous remarks about his older brother. My third son, Brendan, stood by as one of the best men. Kaylin, my only daughter, served as a bridesmaid. As proud parents, my wife, Kathy, and I basked in the good cheer of the gathering.

A lively reception followed under a white sailcloth Sperry Tent decorated with string lights and hanging greenery boxes. White roses held down the centerpieces of the tables.

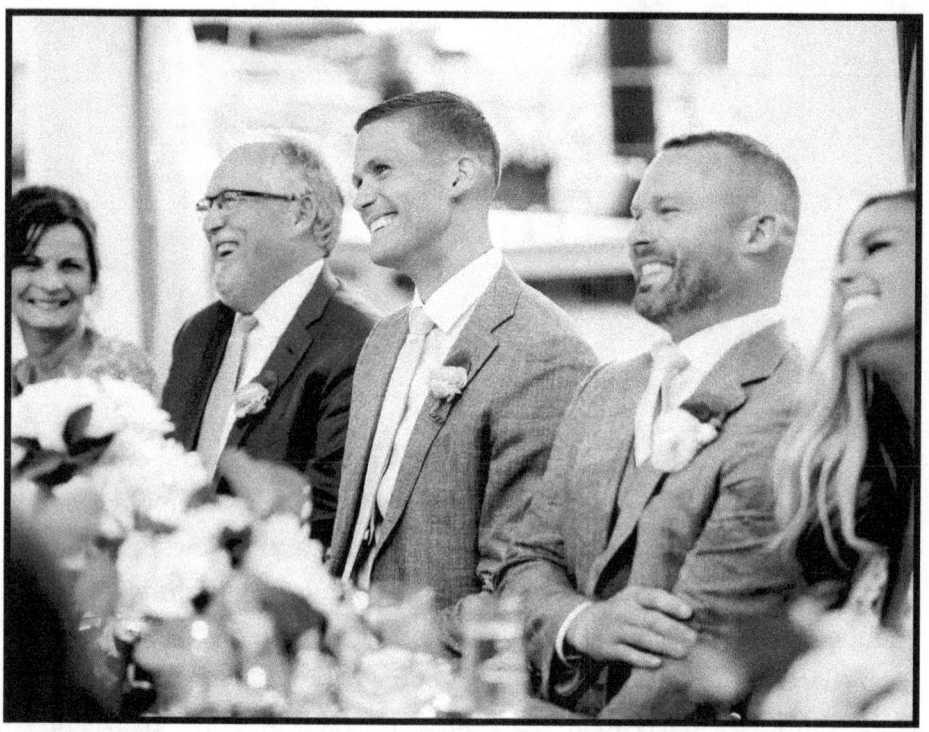

Photo Credit: Melissa Robotti

For the mother-son dance, Dan chose the song "Mother," by Sugarland, which celebrates the unconditional love of a mother. A photograph captured the emotion of the moment, with the two of them beaming at each other.

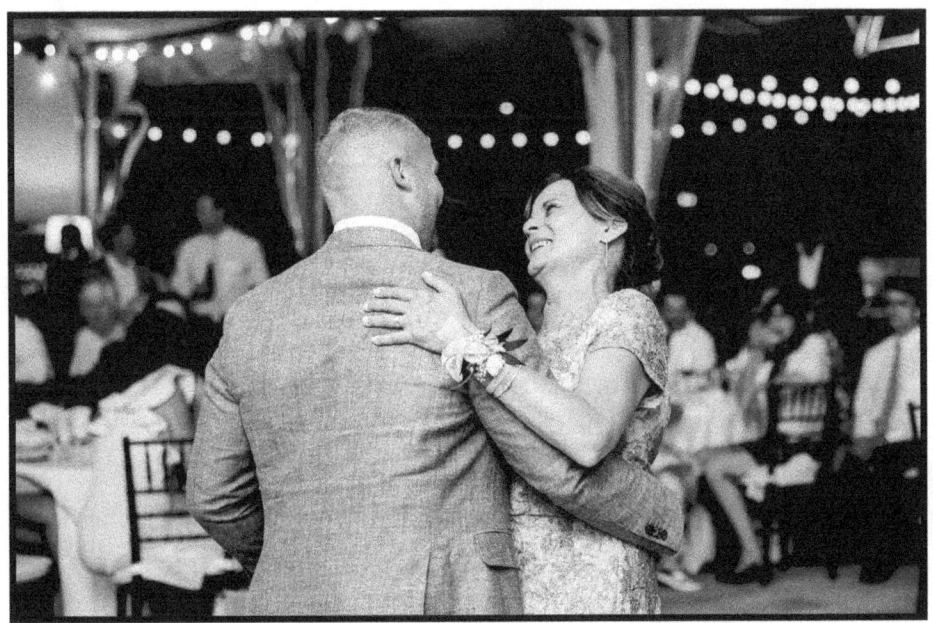

Photo Credit: Melissa Robotti

At various times throughout that day, I took an inventory of how Patrick and his wife, Amanda, were holding up. I saw nothing but relaxed joy and laughter.

But there was also a lingering darkness. Two years before, at age 29 and just a month after marrying Amanda, Patrick was diagnosed with stage 4 colorectal cancer. At the time of Dan's wedding, Patrick was undergoing his 37th round of systemic chemotherapy. The treatment had left him thinner and much less muscular than he had been. His face was slightly gaunt. I knew that he would easily tire and perhaps feel nauseous. It would be easy to lose focus on what was happening around him. As happy as I was 15 months before, when Dan told Kathy and me that he intended to ask his brother to officiate at the ceremony, I had worried whether Patrick's condition would allow him to participate. Far greater was my fear that he might not still be alive.

As his father, a physician and a 14-year survivor of an anomalous advanced stage cancer myself, I could appreciate how Patrick must have felt. All that aside, on that one day, our family could gather in love and happiness, the shadow of Patrick's cancer rendered temporarily invisible.

Patrick was our second child, born on February 9, 1988, in Portland, Maine. At the time, I was a fourth-year medical student, three months away from graduation and starting my postgraduate training at the same hospital where he was born. Beyond Kathy's vigorous pushing, he entered the world without needing any special assistance—no forceps or vacuum extraction device. After delivery and my cutting of the umbilical cord, he was placed on Kathy's upper abdomen.

Almost unnervingly, he looked calm. Even as a newborn, he had a serene and strong presence. He lay there peacefully, not wailing or thrashing in protest of being ejected from the cozy confines of the womb. It didn't take Kathy long to conclude that he was an "old soul." Through infancy and toddlerhood—and unlike Dan, who sometimes reminded us of the Looney Tunes character the Tasmanian Devil—Patrick preferred to sit and watch before taking purposeful action. The need to shed useless frenetic energy was never hardwired in his brain's premotor cortex. And he maintained a steady curiosity.

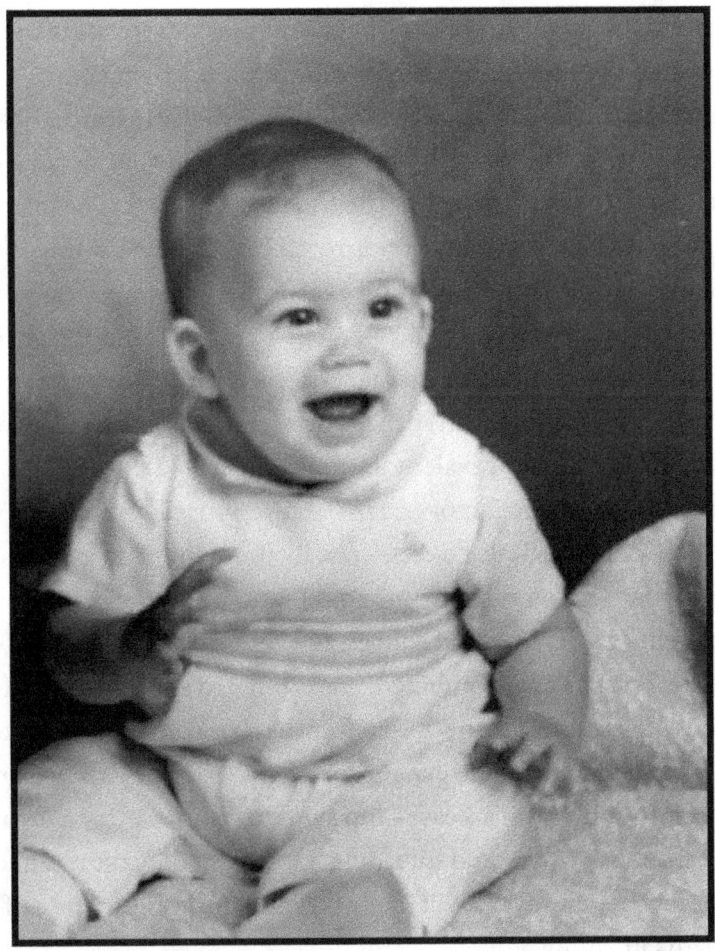

Photo Credit: Kathleen Beauregard

As he got older, Patrick's siblings often called him the "golden child" because of his ability to avoid trouble. Patrick would smirk, but he enjoyed it.

My five happiest days were my wedding day and the births of each of my four children. I vividly recall the moment that Kathy, while sitting at her desk at work, told me she was pregnant with our first child.

But one of the worst days in my life came on September 16, 2017—the day Patrick was diagnosed with stage 4 colorectal cancer. Over my years of seeing patients, I advised scores of people facing catastrophic news, but I never dreamed I would be in that position with my own son.

Colorectal cancer (CRC) is the leading gastrointestinal cancer in Western countries. Historically, it's been a disease that occurs in older adults. For men, the average age at the time of diagnosis is 68; for women, 72. Over the past 20 years, rates of colorectal cancer have declined in people 50 and older. At the same time, however, rates in people under 50 have risen steadily—by an average of 2.2 percent a year in the last three decades. The grim pace seems to be increasing. Forecasts for the upcoming 15 years indicate that breast, gastrointestinal (particularly colorectal), and kidney cancers will be the most prevalent among adults aged 20 to 49.

While multiple risk factors have been proposed, the reason remains unclear. America's industrialized diet—fast food—along with genetics, obesity and the gut microbiome remain among the leading suspects.

In patients with colorectal cancer, the relative five-year survival rates vary by stage. For all stages combined, it is estimated at 68 percent. However, for people with metastatic cancer—cancer that has spread to distant parts of the body—it's 14 percent. The danger for young people is particularly acute because often—as in Patrick's case—no symptoms appear for a decade or so while the cancer is growing and spreading. If the current pattern is unchecked, in the next few decades CRC will likely become the leading cause of cancer-related deaths in young adults.

For decades, national experts in preventive and evidence-based medicine recommended that people at average risk start screening for colon cancer at age 50—typically, by having a colonoscopy. In May 2021, the U.S. Preventive Services Task Force, the American Cancer Society and the National Comprehensive Cancer Network changed their CRC screening guideline to age 45, a suggestion that has come under dispute. (People with a family history of colon cancer or other risk factors should be screened earlier). While it's been well established that detecting CRC precursors—adenomatous polyps—and early-stage disease results in lower mortality rates, screening among Americans lags. Access to screening and patient preferences and acceptance of stool-based tests and/or colonoscopies are contributing factors. A recent paper by the American Cancer Society (ACS) showed that in 2021, only 59 percent of people age 45 and older were screened for colorectal cancer—and only 20 percent of people ages 45–49. (Those numbers remain well below the nationally stated goal of 80 percent). The ACS report also estimated that in 2023, about 153,000 people will be diagnosed with CRC, including 19,550 people under 50; an estimated 3,750 people under 50 will die of the disease. These cases turn inside out the lives of many families, friends and caregivers.

The ACS paper also indicated that the rates of cases of new under-50 CRC—medically known as early-onset colorectal cancer—increased from 11 percent of all cases in 1995 to 20 percent in 2019. It's projected that by the year 2030, one-third of all cases of CRC will occur in people younger than 50. Particularly alarming is the fact that 60 percent of the new cases diagnosed were advanced stage cancers. Again, what's particularly frightening is that in most of these cases, there are no premonitory signs or symptoms. "To date, many early-onset colorectal cancers are detected in emergency rooms, and there are often significant diagnostic delays with this cancer," said Dr. Yin Cao, associate professor of surgery in the public health sciences division at Washington University School of Medicine in St. Louis.

The increase in early-onset CRC reflects an alarming broader trend. Worldwide, health experts report a rise in a range of cancers in younger adults, including breast, prostate, kidney, liver, thyroid and pancreatic cancers. The global rate of early-onset cancer cases rose by nearly 80 percent from 1990 to 2019, while the number of deaths attributed to early-onset cancer also saw an increase of approximately 30 percent. The causes of this general increase are being investigated, with diet, obesity, sleep disruptions, the gut microbiome, environmental pollution and overuse of antibiotics in newborns, children, and adolescents among possible culprits. But it's hard to see how these would have applied to Patrick, who had lived a careful, health-conscious life and whose parents were health-care professionals devoted to nurturing healthy lifestyles for their children.

The Cancer Society's advice is clear: "If there's something you feel that's out of the ordinary, push a little harder for diagnostic tests," said Dr. William Dahut, the chief scientific officer for the ACS. Though Dr. Dahut was speaking specifically about colon cancer, the advice would apply generally to screening for other cancers.

As I write this, I have been a cancer survivor for 18 years. At 49, I was diagnosed with an advanced-stage bladder cancer that typically manifests itself in septuagenarians. Back then, if that cancer showed evidence of regional (local) spread, which mine did, the five-year survival rate was estimated to be 38 percent. Once the shock of learning that I had cancer subsided, the harsh reality of undergoing treatment followed. I went on to endure four cycles of systemic chemotherapy, followed by major surgery. I've lived with the permanent side effects and complications associated with that ever since.

When cancer strikes, everyone in the family is touched. Health care and the family are irrevocably intertwined. Now, my family has been struck twice, and each time, it was like a giant sea swell that slammed us onto a foreign shore, then dragged us tumbling in the backwash that sucked us under. When we finally resurfaced, the undertow always threatened to pull us down again. Cancer became a constant presence in our lives: occupying imaginations, trespassing into memories and infiltrating just about every thought and conversation. Certainty vanished. Questions, mostly unspoken, became the bedrock of family thoughts. *Is Dad going to die? Is Patrick going to die? Am I going to die? How can I help? How can I manage without him? Why did this happen? What else is going to happen? Why...How...When...?*

Perhaps in part because I was adopted, family has always been enormously important to me—always my first priority. In many ways, Kathy and I have been extraordinarily lucky, with four smart, lively, thoughtful kids. Best of all, they loved and enjoyed each other. The laughter that exploded as they chatted and played together often echoes in my mind. Our summer vacations on Cape Cod or The Bahamas, full of swimming, games, cookouts, restaurant dinners and togetherness represent some of my happiest memories. Our family's attendance at the Boston Ballet's annual performance of *The Nutcracker* also provided a rich tradition. As the family grew to include two wonderful daughters-in-law and a terrific son-in-law, the sense of good fun only expanded. My daughter, Kaylin, caught the pleasure we take in each other in an extraordinary essay she wrote as Patrick struggled with his disease. "[W]e make a reservation for nine, and color rushes back to my cheeks," she wrote. "I'm invigorated and full of life at the thought of just being all together."

Despite the harsh reality of what's happened to us over the past 18 or so years, the story at times seemed surreal. Thankfully, our days have been brightened by joyful and seemingly miraculous events—especially three weddings and the births of five grandchildren. I've always been a planner, trying to prepare for whatever comes next. But Kathy wisely reminds me, "All we have is today."

In coping with the traumas of cancer, I've had the advantage of being a doctor. Though sometimes my knowledge and experience gnawed at my sputtering hopes, for the most part my training and connections helped support Patrick and me. I used to wonder how patients with cancer who didn't have experience in health care or access to the best caregivers could understand their illness and all that it entailed. Just navigating the medical maw and the complex decision-making demanded stands as a monumental task. I now have a much deeper understanding of the great distance that separates patients and doctors and how little physicians really understand what their patients are going through, particularly those beset by cancer.

The shortened life expectancy associated with some cancers puts the disease in a different category from, say, diabetes, high blood pressure or heart disease. Physicians who've never had cancer can maintain a degree of hubris that results in underappreciating the enormity of what their patient is experiencing emotionally and physically. Additionally, physicians, like their patients, can be angry at a diagnosis: *Why this person?*

That separation between patients and doctors can include emotional detachment and compartmentalizing of experiences and relationships. I tried to bear that in mind as I resumed my clinical practice after my bout with cancer.

In recounting the cancer journeys that Patrick and I took, I describe complex medical procedures, but I have tried to explain their purposes and put them in language that I hope is accessible to most readers. In that way, I'd like this book to be valuable to people and families facing a cancer diagnosis—a guide to the medical experience and even perhaps a map to help navigate the industrial complex that healthcare delivery has become. If the book doesn't bring solace, perhaps at least it can offer some context and advice.

I'm hopeful also that my experience can serve as a reminder to practicing and aspiring physicians of that distance between doctors and their patients. I realize that the separation sometimes represents a defense mechanism by doctors against the emotional toll of their work. But we can't forget how our behavior—what we say and do—affects the patients we serve who may well be freighted with profound trauma. Between us, Patrick and I dealt with about a dozen doctors, most of whom were wonderfully thoughtful and supportive, but a couple of them needed lessons in human relations.

In addition, I'd like this book to offer insights into how we as a family coped with illness and loss. We all suffered. I made mistakes and regrouped. This account draws from my experience and knowledge, but I've also drawn heavily from conversations with Kathy, as well as conversations with, and written with, and written commentary by, my children.

Patrick and Amanda posted regularly about what they were going through on a website run by CaringBridge, a nonprofit that lets people with illnesses stay in touch with family and friends. Patrick also kept a personal journal that I quote from occasionally.

Patrick and Brendan, who had an especially strong relationship despite an 11-year difference in ages, exchanged letters, confiding in each other in a raw and touching way. Brendan also wrote about tracking the course of his beloved brother's disease. And Kaylin's essay for a creative writing class gives a vivid, sibling-level view of what Patrick and the rest of our family were going through and provides the title for this book.

This book also describes with candor my own emotional pilgrimage. I've learned so much. I've learned that my son was a far better person than I could ever hope to be. As he battled for three years against a debilitating and ultimately deadly disease, he never stopped fighting. If he got knocked down by an ominous setback—by a discouraging scan, for example—he might brood for a few hours or a day, but he inevitably bounced back, ready to fight some more. I still marvel at how he summoned the strength to navigate between acceptance or rejection of his fate. As his prognosis grew gloomier, he turned himself into a vital spokesman for colorectal cancer awareness, giving speeches, providing interviews through assorted media, and making a memorable appearance on *The Today* show. His warnings to young people to get screened have probably saved countless lives.

I've also learned—I'm still learning—how to set aside anger. I was raised a Catholic and Kathy and I brought our family up in the faith, but I had grown almost indifferent over the years. Repeatedly observing good people getting afflicted by horrible illnesses only confirmed that feeling. When cancer struck my son, I raged against God—how could He let this happen? My questions and my fury deepened as I watched Patrick struggle with the disease.

At the very end of his journey, a remarkable woman entered our lives. Mother Olga of the Sacred Heart, a nun who had built a thriving life after growing up in a country where family hardship is commonplace, brought an almost preternaturally powerful sense of love and support to Patrick and our family—something approaching peace. With gentle persuasion, she showed me how to view tragedy and grief through a different lens and restored the little faith I had left.

GEORGE BEAUREGARD

Sir William Osler, a prominent physician-surgeon in the late 19th and early 20th centuries, described cancer in a book's frontispiece as "the emperor of all maladies, the king of all terrors." This book is a family's saga in which the emperor reigned twice. The effect of that lingers. At the center of the story is Patrick Beauregard, whose life journey led him to become a powerful advocate for fighting this disease. What follows is how his and his family's journey played out.

# 2

# The Marine

ONE DAY IN 2013, about 18 months after he graduated from Providence College and while he was working for an electronic medical records company, Patrick came home and asked to speak to Kathy and me. "I'd like to tell you something," he said.

Patrick didn't often make trivial announcements, and so Kathy and I stopped what we were doing and gathered in the family room. My initial thought was that he was about to tell us about a job change.

Instead, he said, "Ever since 9/11 happened, I've felt like I need to do something more meaningful. I'm not saying it's bad, but in general, the way people focus on financial status, job titles, material possessions and what they have and don't have doesn't really mean that much to me. I'm going to enlist in the Marines. I want to pursue a position in intelligence. Like I said, I need to do something that has more meaning for me, like serving my country."

Kathy and I were speechless. As parents of adult children, we have found that there aren't many times when one tells you something important in which he or she doesn't expect advice in return. This was a statement, with no advice sought. As remarkable and out-of-the-blue as the news was, my heart swelled with pride and admiration for our then-25-year-old son. Still, I immediately worried, as did Kathy, about a potential deployment to Afghanistan.

Our family didn't have multi-generational military roots. Both of Patrick's grandfathers had served in the armed forces during the Korean War, though neither had seen combat. That notwithstanding, Patrick had been interested in hearing about their experiences. Shortly after the 1998 release of *Saving Private Ryan*, the iconic movie that opens with the Normandy invasion, I took Dan and Patrick to a screening. Dan was interested, but Patrick—then around ten—was riveted. He was similarly fascinated with the HBO miniseries *Band of Brothers*, a dramatized account of the exploits of a parachute infantry battalion of the U.S. Army during World War II. The acclaimed series debuted two days before the 9/11 attacks. Later, after Kathy and I had visited Normandy on a French vacation, Patrick drilled me with questions.

Unexpected as his announcement was, it didn't stun me that this was something he would do. In his quiet, determined way, Patrick always seemed to expect more of himself. For all his boyish charm, he intended to lead his life with a larger purpose.

Patrick had been an excellent student. After a year at our local public high school in Medfield, Massachusetts, he asked if he could join Dan at Thayer Academy, a private school in Braintree, Massachusetts. He started there as a freshman and did well academically while playing varsity basketball and lacrosse. A skilled lacrosse defenseman, he was big, strong, fast and had good footwork and stick work. Accordingly, he was frequently urged to cross the midfield line and become a "middie"—an offensive player. He preferred defense. Chippy opponents often regretted antagonizing Patrick.

At Providence College, a Catholic school in Providence, Rhode Island, he particularly enjoyed several international politics courses and graduated with a Bachelor of Science in political science degree in 2011. During his sophomore year, a mutual friend introduced him to another Providence student, Amanda Jane Flood, who was majoring in political science and economics. Amanda grew up with her parents and two younger sisters in Lowell, about 30 miles northwest of Boston. Her ambition was to become a lawyer, and following her graduation summa cum laude from Providence, she enrolled at Suffolk University Law School, in Boston.

As the relationship between Amanda and Patrick deepened and a future together seemed inevitable, friends and family joined their names and started calling the pair "Panda." The cuteness of the name notwithstanding, they were a power couple.

Kathy and I supported Patrick's decision to join the Marines, though warily, given the state of the world. Because of his deepening relationship with Amanda, Patrick chose reserve duty which, after ten weeks of basic training, represents an eight-year commitment: four years in monthly weekend drills and two-week summer duty, followed by four years in the individual ready reserve (IRR). Meantime, he could continue with a civilian job. Despite multiple attempts by the local USMC recruiter to have Patrick enlist before the intelligence position he wanted was available, Patrick deferred. After a seven-month wait, the position opened in the fall of 2013, and he enlisted. His training site was the famously rigorous Parris Island base in Beaufort County, South Carolina.

Patrick was generally buttoned-up about his Marine experience—after all, he was in intelligence—but he did tell us something about the training, which was eye-opening for a non-military family like ours. When the time came, he and other recruits flew from Boston's Logan International Airport to Charleston, South Carolina. From there, they boarded a bus and began the 80-mile drive to Parris Island. Patrick described the ride as extraordinary: On orders, the recruits spent more than half the journey seated with their heads between their knees, looking at the floor. (That was the first introduction to following orders, he explained, and was deliberately done to disorient the recruits).

GEORGE BEAUREGARD

Shortly after arrival at the depot, the recruits were allowed one phone call. A drill instructor was stationed next to the phone, ready to intervene if any conversation turned rogue. Patrick stood in a long line, waiting for his turn to call home and recite a scripted message. Kathy answered his call. "Hi, family," he said over considerable background noise. "Just want to let you know that I've arrived. Everything is okay. I have to go now." The next sound Kathy heard was a click. Over the course of the next ten weeks, we received eight short letters from Private Beauregard, talking mostly about training. No other communication.

He later told us a bit about the last, most grueling test that recruits endure—the so-called Crucible—a 54-hour exercise comprising eight major training events designed to test the mental, physical and moral capabilities of the recruits. Under sleep-deprived conditions, the test requires teamwork to accomplish specific tasks. The Crucible ends with the recruits taking a demanding nine-mile night march to the base's Iwo Jima Memorial, where they are awarded the eagle, globe and anchor insignia and become Marines.

Thanksgiving and Christmas are important events in our house, particularly to Kathy. Patrick's absence that year created a void in the family that we knew was temporary but left us feeling less than whole. In late January 2014, Kathy and I, along with Amanda, Kaylin, Dan and Brendan traveled to Parris Island for Patrick's graduation, an elaborate ceremony featuring precise marching and formations. When the new Marines were finally dismissed, we all had turns embracing him. He looked tired and much thinner than the last time we had seen him. But he was flashing a huge smile.

Patrick came home for a ten-day leave before more training in Virginia, Massachusetts, and San Diego. Then he continued as a reservist, with its weekend and summer obligations, eventually rising to the rank of lance corporal. Although it nearly happened once, he was never mobilized for active duty. He told us nothing about his intelligence work.

RESERVATIONS FOR NINE

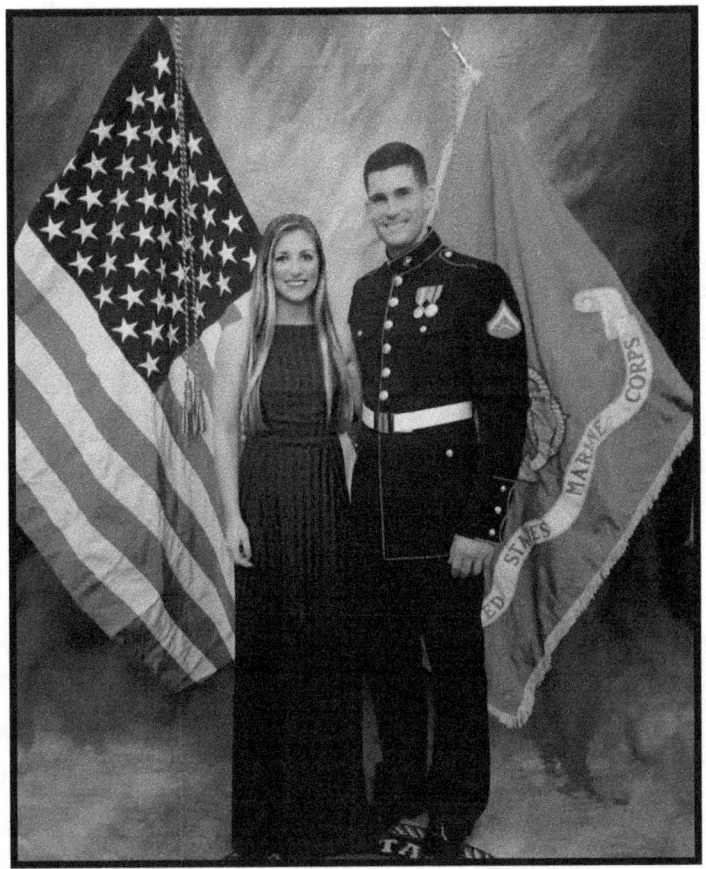

Photo Credit: Sonny Bui

In some ways, the situation resembled what a close friend of mine had experienced over many years with his son in the CIA. My friend almost never knew exactly what his son did or where he was stationed. Months would go by without any contact.

Patrick was proud of his service, but I suspect that the experience was not all he had hoped. Later, while battling his cancer, he said several times in his private journal that he wished he could have done more for his country.

He stored his unloaded Marine Reserve weapons in our house, which caused a minor trauma when Kathy found him letting Brendan handle the guns.

By then, Patrick had landed a job with Northeast Security Solutions, a leading full-service security outfit based in Westwood, Massachusetts, and covering New England. The company provides alarms and safes, as well as surveillance, intelligence and technology services. Patrick quickly rose through the ranks to become an assistant vice president of operations.

Amanda's career as a lawyer started with her joining a law firm in Boston, where her focus was on Massachusetts and federal regulatory compliance in health care.

With Patrick and Amanda both embarked on their careers, they started living together in an apartment in South Boston. On the third floor, the apartment was small but afforded a great view of the Boston skyline. On a cold night in February 2016, while standing in front of South Boston's famed Dorchester Heights Monument, which commemorates an important American victory in the Revolutionary War, Patrick proposed to Amanda, and she accepted.

Amanda joined us several times for our summer vacation in Chatham, a town on the elbow of Cape Cod known for its pristine beaches, tidal shoals and fleeting sandbars. She decided that she wanted the wedding ceremony held there.

Patrick was the first of our children to marry. The wedding was held August 18, 2017, in Holy Redeemer Church in Chatham. White hydrangeas, blush spray roses and eucalyptus adorned the front pews. The wedding party included 19 people. Dan and Brendan were co-best men and Kaylin was one of the bridesmaids. Amanda's sisters, Regan and Devin, were the co-maids of honor. Around 150 people attended.

Patrick and Amanda stood in front of an altar covered by a white cloth, two lighted candles and a liturgical book. Amanda looked elegant and beautiful in her white wedding gown. Patrick posed as the straight-backed Marine beside her. They were the picture of a couple full of promise and life.

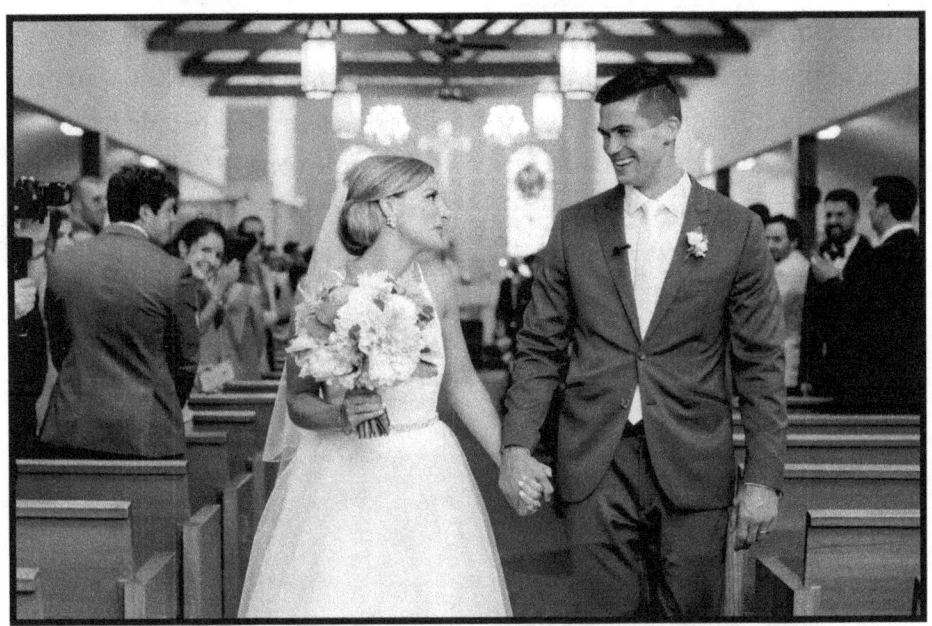

Photo Credit: Kelly Cronin Bicknell

A reception followed at the Chatham Bars Inn, a venerable beachfront resort overlooking Pleasant Bay. Except for a brief, ill-timed shower, the sun shone brightly in the summer sky. Their wedding song was "Sweetest Devotion," by Adele. Patrick and Amanda were not prone to public displays of their emotions. But watching them dance together during those moments provided me with a clear view of their powerful connection.

During toasts, Amanda's father, Charlie Flood, spoke of being "deeply proud of our Amanda Panda Bear." He told Patrick that as the father of three girls, "I couldn't be happier to finally have some male backup." He blessed the couple: "May you grow old together and may the love you feel this day grow in your hearts forever."

Following dinner and the bouquet toss, the dancing began. Like Patrick, Amanda's manner was usually restrained. But when the song "Ironic," by Alanis Morissette came up, Amanda raced into the middle of a circling crowd. Holding her gown up off the floor, she danced flamboyantly and sang along at the top of her voice. When Patrick joined her, it was like watching an electric arc, seeing these two normally self-controlled people let loose.

For the mother-son dance, Patrick chose the song "93 Million Miles," by Jason Mraz. While the song title describes the Earth's distance from the sun, it lyrically and warm-heartedly speaks to one's ability, regardless of their location, to return home.

A photo of Kathy and Pat taken during the dance shows him calmly gazing at her as she gazed back with her palms gently touching his cheeks.

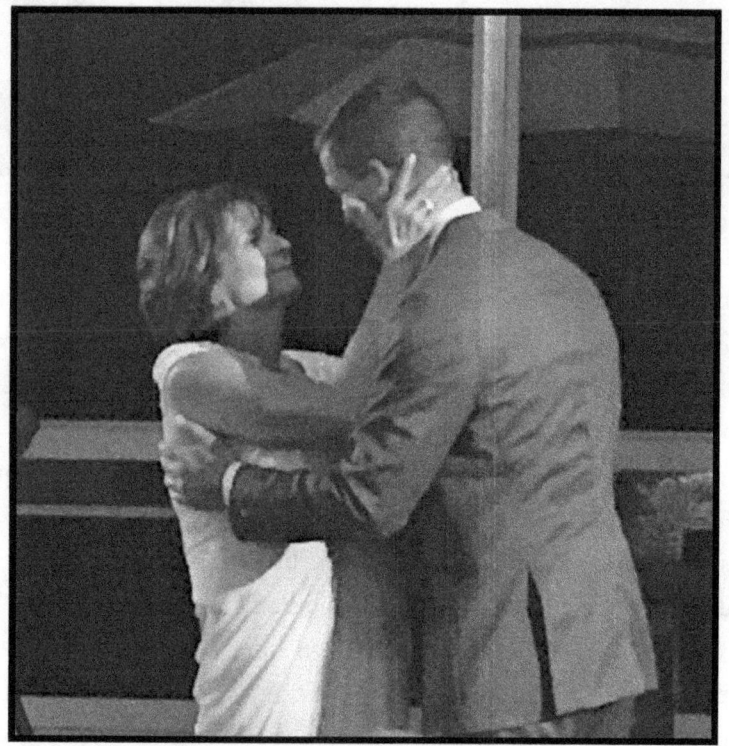

Photo Credit: Kelly Cronin Bicknell

The following day, we hosted a family cookout at our vacation rental in Chatham. It ended with Patrick and Amanda driving off to their apartment in South Boston to prepare for their flight to San Francisco and then on to the French Polynesian islands of Tahiti and Bora Bora. Knowing that Patrick's primary bond was now with Amanda, Kathy made a mother's wish that her child had found someone who would love him as much as she did.

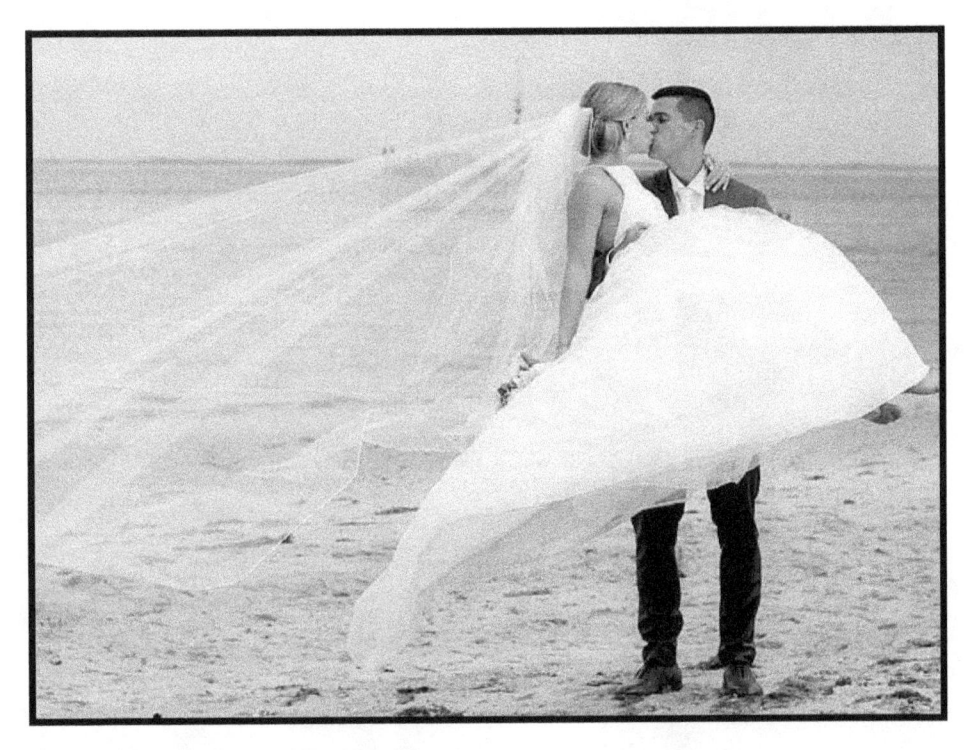

Photo Credit: Kelly Cronin Bicknell

The delighted couple set off for the sandy white beaches, and their friends and family felt certain they were destined for a long and joyful life together. Yet, unbeknownst to us all, Patrick's body had already betrayed him.

# 3

# Misbehaving Cells

BACTERIA ARE UNICELLULAR organisms and humans are obviously multicellular ones. The human body consists of about 37 trillion specialized cells that, among other things, construct a diverse ensemble of 78 unique organs that comprise 13 different interconnected systems, including the cardiovascular, gastrointestinal, musculoskeletal, nervous, endocrine, and other systems. These systems, much like orchestras and ballet companies, typically function harmoniously to maintain a steady state while responding to various external stimuli. However, the complexity of being multicellular also presents the (perhaps inevitable) risk of genomic instability, leading to such issues as cancer.

Fundamentally, cancer is a disease of genes. Aging, oxidative metabolism—how cells use oxygen to turn food into energy—and replication errors constantly occur in human cells. Research has shown that most cancer-causing mutations arise by chance, while high-risk, inherited genetic mutations are rare, leading to a belief that the majority of cancers are largely unavoidable.

Various epigenetic processes, affected by both environmental and behavioral factors, have been identified as being natural, and crucial for the proper functioning of many organs. These processes can alter gene activity without changing the genetic sequence. However, if these processes occur incorrectly, they can result in numerous adverse health consequences.

The specific three-dimensional shapes of proteins and nucleic acids, known as tertiary structures, are created through the folding and cross-linking of polypeptide chains. These chains are the fundamental building blocks of proteins and amino acids, essential for the existence of life. The tertiary structure plays a crucial role in determining the unique function and interactions of proteins.

Among others, two epigenetic processes in human cancer are well known: methylation, the addition of a methyl group—3 hydrogen atoms and 1 carbon atom—to a DNA molecular target, and acetylation, which modifies the chromatin structure—a mixture of DNA and proteins that form chromosomes—and influence gene expression. Tightly coiled chromatin tends to be nonfunctional—not to be expressed—, while more open chromatin is expressed and functional. Not all genes are active at all times. At any given time, we are using only about 1 percent of our genetic material; the rest of it is in an "off" mode. Methylation is how the body turns off "bad" genes. But not all methylation leads to beneficial outcomes.

As individuals age, specific DNA regions in cells of the colon tend to have increased methylation. This process can affect gene expression and regulate various biological functions within cells.

But certain factors such as a poor (Western) diet, sedentary lifestyle, stress and environmental exposures, can keep bad genes active.

Even in normal cells, spontaneous genetic mutations can occasionally occur. The majority of these mutations are harmless and have minimal to no impact, while some may even have advantageous effects. On the other hand, some harmful mutations are the result of inherited abnormalities, while others are caused by external factors, such as tobacco or chemicals.

In Patrick, as in most patients who develop cancer, it probably started meekly as a lone gene in a cell that became the victim of a spontaneous, random mistake in its DNA—like a typo. Given how long it takes colorectal cancers to go from single cells to small tumors and to large invasive neoplasms, the mutation probably ignited when Patrick was in his late teens, a strong and active young athlete.

In Patrick's case, there's no evidence that either an inheritance or a toxic environmental substance was the cause. That's where the random typo comes in, disrupting the cell's normal business of coding for proteins involved in cell multiplication and growth. Its programming altered, the cell misunderstood its previous instructions and started to misbehave, while still sitting on the inner lining of Patrick's colon.

Over time, new theories and discoveries about the nature of cancer's origin and its behavior have continued to emerge and evolve.

Since James Watson and Francis Crick's groundbreaking discovery of its double helical structure in 1953, the DNA in our chromosomes has been seen as the blueprint and instruction manual for life, with gene regulation processes executing the plan. Genes were once thought to have "on" and "off" switches, similar to light fixtures, computers, and televisions. However, current thinking on gene regulation has shifted away from the idea of a firm, selective process towards a belief that it may be more lackadaisical, aggregated and indifferent to its molecular surroundings.

Tumor growth is now viewed as unhinged development rather than a simple overindulgence of replication. This new perspective has led some researchers to describe cancer as a "disease of organization" rather than just a disease of cells, moving away from the traditional concept of a cancer cell.

During autopsies, a significant number of men who have not been clinically diagnosed with prostate cancer are discovered to have the disease. It is challenging to comprehend—and accept—that it is a likely part of the human condition to have cancer cells present,—whether or not there are detectable signs of cancer. This concept is similar to such age-related conditions as presbyopia, presbycusis, and skin spots.

Recent advances in cellular and genomic analytics technology have shown that tumors consist of a variety of cell types, including healthy cells organized in a more structured manner resembling organs rather than a chaotic mass of rapidly reproducing cells. This suggests that cancer may not be a result of malfunction, but rather a shift to a different, more organized lifestyle having a plan. Dr. Siddartha Mukherjee, a renowned oncologist and researcher has stated that cancer is not just a disruption of normal cell development leading to uncontrollable growth.

Another problem stems from the fact that the healthy cells in a tumor are not merely innocent bystanders—some actually aid the cancer cells in their malicious actions.

The long held and accepted proposed model of CRC development—the so-called adenoma-carcinoma cascade—has it occurring over a span of 5 to 10 years, during which mutations occur in an adenomatous polyp, leading it to become a malignant tumor.

At the molecular level, CRC results largely from the accretion of modifications—based on genetic factors and environmental and behavioral influences—in the cells on the thin tissue lining the colon. More recently, researchers have discovered that, perhaps, cancer is a disease wherein a mutated gene sits dormant until it's activated by something in its environment or an external catalyst barges in and sets the cancer cells in motion.

An unanswered question looms large: Do early-onset colorectal cancers diverge from that classical pathway and develop faster?

The thought that Patrick perhaps had either a healthy tissue environment that was primed for tumor development or an inherent genomic instability—something that lay hidden until being coaxed to expose itself and do its malicious work by something else—was frightening.

Cancer cells divide wildly and create misbehaving copies of themselves. In Patrick's case, the cancerous mass eventually became big enough to penetrate the four layers of his sigmoid colon, including finally the serosa, the outermost layer.

Cancer cells that breach the serosa can spread to nearby lymph nodes, thus potentially spreading further through the lymphatic system—a pathway for travel throughout the body. In addition, as cancer cells grow, they need more blood to bring them oxygen and other nutrients, so they signal the tumor to make new blood vessels, opening additional routes for the cancer to travel. Metastasis—the term used when cancer cells spread to different parts of the body—is an incongruous mix of meta and stasis: "beyond stillness" in Latin.

A review published in the International Journal of Sciences in 2021 estimated that more than 300,000 people would receive a new diagnosis of metastatic cancer upon initial evaluation during that year.

Metastatic cancer, in short, is the travel biology of cancer cells. And one in which different oncogenes—mutated genes that can cause cancer—can exist in the different sites of spread.

The human immune system has a function termed immunosurveillance, whereby foreign and abnormal cells can be recognized and abolished, so in the earliest stages of cancer formation, the body's immune system eliminates certain individual cancer cells as they arise. Therefore, cancer cells must escape detection by the immune system for the tumor to spread and grow.

As these cells expand, they become clever at evading the immune system. In some instances, they alter their surface and become unrecognizable; in others, they produce chemicals or signals that neutralize immune cells. In some ways, cancer cells adapt better and grow faster than normal human cells. In their drive for life, you might say cancer cells are idealized versions of ourselves.

Most patients with cancer do not die from the growth of the primary tumor, but from the profoundly harmful effects that metastasis imposes on many vital physiological functions—referred to as cancer "swamp gas" by a physician researcher. In the end, the human body can only take so much before reaching a breaking point. A sobering reality is that metastatic cancer kills 10 million people a year—and is essentially incurable.

That notwithstanding, the malevolent, aggressive, and harmful new species that began on the inner lining of Patrick's colon grew and spread, eventually colonizing his lungs and lymph nodes. All the while, he had an active athletic career, went through Marine training, worked hard, fell in love, and celebrated his marriage with no sign that anything was amiss—until those cancer cells announced their presence with terrifying clarity.

# 4

# Opening Acts

CONSIDER MY LIFE as a play. I entered the drama in Act 1 but wasn't given the script and therefore didn't know my lines. Act 1 started with my adoptive parents, Rodolphe (Rudy) and Marguerite (Peggy) Beauregard losing their newborn first child, a daughter, after a traumatic labor and delivery. The resulting damage left Peggy infertile.

But their desire to have children persisted. So, they investigated adoption, hiring a social services agency, the Catholic Charities of Boston. They requested a girl. But during one of their visits to the agency, the nuns told them that, although no girls were available, they had two 18-month-old identical twin boys—who had been cycled between five foster homes since birth—to show them. A nun escorted my brother, Gary, and me into the room. After spending a short period with us, my mother looked at my father and said, "I can't leave without them." My father raised concerns about the challenges of suddenly having two toddlers whom they didn't know. My mother was resolute.

The adoption process began and weeks later, Rudy and Peg brought Gary and me to their home, in Bellingham, Massachusetts, a small, blue-collar town on the southwestern fringe of metropolitan Boston and abutting the old mill town of Woonsocket, Rhode Island. My brother and I shared a room on the second floor, across from my new parents' bedroom. My paternal grandparents lived in the house behind us. Several other extended-family members also lived close by. They pitched in to help my father build the home we later moved to nearby in Bellingham.

About the time that my brother and I were six, Rudy and Peg told us that we were adopted, which enhanced the trust and affection we felt for our adoptive parents. I've never known the identity of my biological parents, and I've learned nothing about my life before Gary and I came to live with Rudy and Peg.

It's well known that tremendous brain development occurs during very early childhood. In the first year of life, more than a million neural connections are made every second. Concurrently, massive overproduction takes place of synapses, the transmitters of nerve impulses that run the nervous system. This is followed by a gradual reduction of synapses. That pruning, which is highly experience-dependent and defined by genetic and environmental interactions, determines largely how the brain develops. Pathways activated by experience are strengthened while ones that go unused are eliminated—use it or lose it. Repetitive and familiar everyday routines play a major role. Character and behavior are fine-tuned and moderated as needed.

Given the neuroscience, I am certain that whatever happened during my first 18 months—while my brain was under construction, expanding and trimming—influenced my hardwiring and shaped how I became me.

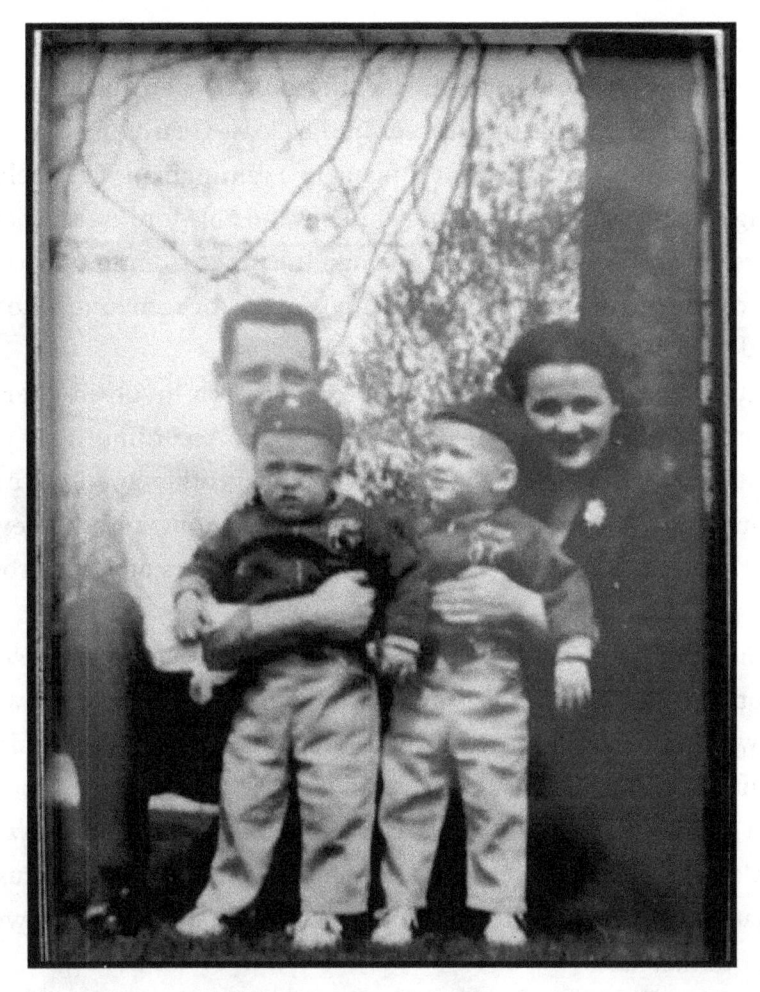

Photo Credit: Ernest R. Beauregard

Neither Rudy nor Peg had finished high school. My mother was one of 13 children and was needed at home to look after the family. My father grew up in West Warwick, Rhode Island, the son of a textile worker. Years later, his mother was diagnosed with lymphoma—cancer in the lymph nodes—and refused treatment, dying at 65. As cancer was generally considered a highly stigmatized disease then, and not often openly discussed, I never learned much about my grandmother's illness.

## GEORGE BEAUREGARD

Before his 18th birthday, my father enlisted in the U.S. Coast Guard. During his four years of service, he met my mother, who quickly dissuaded him from pursuing a full-time career in the Coast Guard. Instead, he took a job at the General Motors auto plant in Framingham, Massachusetts, working on the part of the assembly line responsible for inserting engines into cars. Over the years, he rose through the ranks from line worker to a quality control manager—quite an achievement for someone who hadn't finished high school.

My dad worked at GM for 32 years. His job involved alternating six-month periods of working days, then nights. Accordingly, my parents were often apart during the evenings when my brother and I were home. For many years, my mother was a stay-at-home mom, and she never got a driver's license. Later, she worked for several years at A.T. Cross, the famous pen company.

The household was happy, though low-key. My mom was lively and affectionate—she told Kathy while I was courting her that her two sons "lived within, not under, my heart." My dad had a remarkable talent for fixing just about anything. I can't recall a single time when a repair man came to our home. Dad could replace toilets and sinks, fix lawn mowers and snow blowers, put up fences and do other assorted odd jobs. (It frustrated him that I wasn't inclined to do the same). Money was tight, but we lived within our means.

As practicing Catholics, we attended church every Sunday and went to all the Catholic holiday services but weren't devout. Through eighth grade, my brother and I attended a Catholic elementary school, Assumption School in Bellingham, and we served as altar boys during some of those years. Because we were apt pupils, Mount St. Charles, a prominent Catholic high school in Woonsocket, offered us a 50-percent discount on tuition to enroll there. I wanted to go, but my parents couldn't afford even the discounted tuition, so Gary and I attended Bellingham High School.

Catholicism didn't really come alive to me until just after high school, when I got involved with a Catholic youth organization based in Woonsocket. I joined primarily to play on the basketball and baseball teams, but that led to participating in a spiritual activity known as Monday Night Faith Talk and Mass. On those nights, young adults came together to listen to a timely talk about the Catholic faith. Hearing others speak about the challenges that were testing their faith, and how the power of community and prayer helped them through difficult times resonated with me. But after a couple of years, work and school started to keep me too busy, and I stopped participating.

Throughout our childhood and up to the eighth grade, Gary and I were mostly called "the twins," without our names. We shared a single bedroom and dressed much the same. We shared friends. Beyond finding it occasionally annoying, I didn't give it much thought. We were usually inseparable. Upon entering high school, however, our willingness to navigate in that closely shared space started to decline. We started wearing different clothes, listening to different music, reading different sorts of books, playing different sports and having different friends. I didn't fully recognize then how much we were drifting apart.

The separation dramatically manifested itself one day when I heard Gary scream to our parents during an argument, "I didn't ask you to adopt me!" Enraged, I yelled, "How dare you say that? You ungrateful piece of shit!" I started pummeling him. My mother and father had to separate us. From that moment on, our sibling relationship was profoundly changed. In hindsight, I realized that anger about the whole "identical twin" thing had been simmering within my brother over the years. We pretty much went our separate ways.

Shortly after he graduated from high school, Gary shocked us by announcing that he was gay. It was 1974. Most people's understanding and acceptance of homosexuality wasn't what it is now. But my parents were accepting and didn't love him any less.

GEORGE BEAUREGARD

Gary and I were both going to attend Bridgewater State College, in Bridgewater, Massachusetts, but just as the first semester was about to start in September 1974, he surprised us again by announcing that he didn't want to go there. Instead, he got a job at a Bancroft tennis racket plant in Woonsocket. A couple of years later, he enrolled at the University of Massachusetts at Amherst and graduated with a Bachelor of Science degree in psychology. I visited him at college only once during his four years there. Following his graduation, he worked in Boston as a counselor for Larry Kramer, the famous AIDS activist who founded ACT UP, a movement to fight governmental indifference to AIDS.

I earned high honors from Bellingham High and wanted to go to Harvard. My parents, however, felt that being co-signers for my student loans was a risk they couldn't afford, so I enrolled at Bridgewater State College as a biology major. As it turned out, the far-from-challenging academic environment in Bellingham left me with poor study habits. At the end of my freshman year at Bridgewater State, my GPA was 1.9. Embarrassed, I withdrew.

I got a job at the same Bancroft factory where my brother had worked (and I helped make a few rackets later used by Bjorn Borg). But it took only about six months for me to decide that I needed to go back to college. One day, while perusing a Rhode Island Junior College catalog, I came across the associate degree program in radiologic technology, a program that trained people to become X-ray technicians. I applied and was accepted. I had to pay for college myself, so I worked three to four nights a week at a bar and grill. But failure is often the greatest teacher, and I completed the two years of study with a 4.0 GPA.

One day during college, a female classmate turned to me and said, "I know the perfect person for you." I was skeptical, but the classmate added, "She's very pretty and really smart." Her friend, Kathy, was in the physical therapy program at Simmons College, a prestigious, private women's school in Boston. Kathy insisted that we meet in a group setting, so, one night, we separately arrived for dinner with several others at a Ground Round restaurant in Providence. When the evening started, we were at opposite ends of a long table. As the night passed, I made my way to sit next to her. We talked about everything. To my delight, she agreed to see me again.

Kathy had grown up with her parents and two younger sisters in affluent Barrington, Rhode Island—a far cry from my roots in blue-collar Bellingham. While T-shirts and blue jeans were the customary attire of my neighbors and classmates, many Barrington residents followed the Newport style of pink button-down collared shirts and green khaki pants.

I had to up my game (if not my wardrobe). My mother implored me, "Don't lose her. She's very special. Girls like her don't come along frequently." I knew she was right. I proposed to Kathy on Christmas Day in 1980, and on May 16, 1982, we stood at the altar in St. Luke's Church in Barrington and exchanged marriage vows. I saw nothing in my new wife's eyes but a future filled with happiness.

We first lived in a one-bedroom apartment in Walpole, Massachusetts. By then, I was working at a small community hospital in Woonsocket. Following her Simmons graduation, magna cum laude, in December 1981, Kathy went to work as an inpatient staff physical therapist at Mount Auburn Hospital in Cambridge, Massachusetts. Our careers in healthcare had begun. Later, she took a job at the hospital where I worked and we moved to a second-floor apartment in Lincoln, Rhode Island.

The duties of a hospital-based X-ray tech include providing services in the main department as well as the emergency and operating rooms and the intensive-care unit. The experience fueled my ambition to become a doctor. When time permitted, rather than sit in the tech lounge and chat, I lingered with the department radiologists, the specialists who interpret medical images generated by radiographs. I would listen as they reviewed the clinical context for the test order, images and dictated reports.

In the emergency room, I befriended one of the attending physicians, Wayne Larson. I shared with him my ambition to become a doctor. He asked the key question: "Why?"

"Because I know that if I never try, I'm going to spend the rest of my life thinking about it with regret."

He smiled broadly. "That's the best reason to go for it. I'll be more than happy to serve as a reference for you if you need one."

Hearing that, I bolted out of the starting block. With only an associate degree, I went to school several nights a week to fulfill the premed course requirements. I was accepted at the University of New England College of Osteopathic Medicine, in Biddeford, Maine. Then 28, I began my studies in July 1984 and Kathy landed a full-time faculty position in the university's physical therapy program.

Before we moved to Maine, my mother, then in her early fifties, developed uterine cancer. Her treatment consisted of major surgery and radiation. Despite the typical side effects, she never complained through her ordeal.

Given my mother's situation, I informed her that I would defer my enrollment in medical school for a year. Her response was firm. "Absolutely not. This is an opportunity that not many people get. You've earned it. You will be a great doctor. I'll be fine. Everything will be okay."

A few weeks after her surgery, both of her legs swelled up. Her oncologist didn't recognize that this probably indicated the presence of a blood clot. While at home one night, she developed acute chest pain, shortness of breath and then collapsed in the bathroom. Distraught, my father called 911 and then me. She was taken to Woonsocket Hospital, where Kathy and I worked, and we immediately headed there. When I raced through the ER doors, I saw the shock and dismay on the faces of those staffing the ER that night. The doctor on duty was Wayne Larson. "I'm so sorry, George," he said and began to cry.

Once I became a physician, I realized that her death—which was caused by a pulmonary embolism—had probably been preventable. It was a failure to diagnose.

Going through medical school is intellectually stimulating and arduous. The high demands of the academic studies primarily fall during the first 24 to 30 months. In total, classroom, lab and studying time consumed about 12 hours a day. To limit notetaking chores, students in my class served as scribes on a rotating basis; copies of the notes were then made available to the rest of the class. (The same system held true for the coffee urn service, as medical students drink a lot of coffee).

In essence, going through medical school is really just about memorizing loads of information. That said, true learning kicks in during clinical rotations, internships, and residency, where you deal with real people, the countless variations about how illnesses and disease manifest themselves, and the everyday challenges that doctors face.

The curriculum started with such basic medical concepts as biochemistry and neuroanatomy (by far the hardest courses), embryology, histology and immunology. Courses about the structure and functions of the human body (anatomy and physiology) followed. No student forgets dissecting a cadaver in a basement anatomy lab. It seems as if the smell of formaldehyde stays with you for months. The study of diseases, diagnoses and treatment concepts followed. At the time, there was only one course on medical ethics and humanities. Years three and four consisted of clinical clerkships, mostly in states outside of Maine.

As a medical student, anatomy and physiology were what I loved—how organs, particularly the heart and the brain, are structured and how they function normally and when afflicted by disease. The other material really didn't resonate with me. I viewed it rather as I felt about higher mathematics—stuff to memorize to pass an exam. I would feel very differently about my notions and biases years later.

## GEORGE BEAUREGARD

The average age of my first-year class was 28, several years older than the national medical school average of 24. Like me, many of my classmates had prior careers in such medical fields as pharmacology, exercise physiology, psychology and nursing. But other students had worked as artists, teachers and business people. While nationally, many medical students exhibit stress and symptoms of anxiety and depression, I didn't see much of that in our class of 68. Maturity matters. (That's not to say some weird behavior didn't happen occasionally).

Like me, many students were married, so symptoms of social isolation didn't appear common among my classmates. Kathy and I became friends with some of my classmates and their spouses: Some lived in our apartment complex. One classmate, an aspiring obstetrician/gynecologist from northern Maine, lived with us for several months. For me, sleep deprivation really didn't become an issue until my post-graduate training.

During the four years, Kathy enjoyed her position as part of the physical therapy faculty. Her paycheck was small, but it provided enough money (barely) to cover our living expenses. Student loans funded my annual tuition bills.

Our first son, Dan, arrived when I was a second-year student. His delivery came shortly after midnight on April 1, 1986, after a labor of more than 24 hours. A very active child from the start, he was walking by nine months. Patrick followed during my fourth year, three months before my graduation.

Kathy was mostly a single parent during those times. Dan went to an on-campus daycare program, but trying to balance childcare and her job was sometimes stressful for her. But four years passed, and we each usually handled things well.

Sometime during her cancer treatment, my mother had implored me prophetically, "Look after your brother—he's going to need you to steady him." In early 1986, Gary gave us terrible news. He'd been diagnosed with the so-called acquired immunodeficiency syndrome (AIDS). In December of that year, he was recruited by the National Institutes of Health (NIH) in Bethesda, Maryland, to participate in a clinical trial. The objective was to find if a patient with AIDS would benefit from receiving a transplant of stem cells from the patient's identical twin or a close relation. The stem cells would be taken from blood in the arms and harvested directly from bone marrow in my pelvis.

When Gary asked if I was willing to serve as a donor, Dan was eight months old. Back then, much remained unknown about the transmission of the virus. Kathy and I worried about the potential impact of casual contact with Gary. Still, I remembered what my mother had asked—to look over my brother—, and I felt a treatment like this might save Gary's life.

I agreed and Gary went ahead with the trial. (During one of the clinic visits, Kathy and I met Dr. Anthony Fauci, who was running AIDS research at the National Institutes of Health). For me, the procedures went without complications. Although I never read any official publication about the trial results, I later learned that the trial showed no significant effects from the transplantation procedure.

Over the next year or so, Gary suffered respiratory failure due to pneumonia, from which he recovered, and various other AIDS-related opportunistic infections that sapped his life. Dr. Jerome Groopman, one of the world's leading AIDS researchers, helped care for him.

A few days before his death, I visited Gary in his apartment, in Boston. I wasn't prepared for what I saw. He had a cachectic appearance—his body had wasted terribly. He was bed-bound and had a blank stare. His speech, barely a whisper, was at times, incoherent. Gary seemed to fluctuate between sleep and wakefulness as I sat by his bed, desperately trying to manufacture words that would provoke memories and be meaningful to him.

In some ways, I suppose, I was trying to repair in a day the estranged relationship we had suffered over the years. I have no idea if anything I said achieved that. As I drove back to Maine, I knew that it was probably the last time I would see him alive. To this day, I can't escape the feeling that I didn't do enough to bring our relationship back to where it was when we were boys. On December 3, 1987, his significant other phoned. Gary had passed away comfortably, surrounded by friends. As he wished, he was cremated, and his ashes placed alongside our adoptive mother at the St. Jean-Baptiste Cemetery in Bellingham.

The only solace I could feel was that my mother didn't have to endure the death of a son.

In 1987, AIDS took 13,448 lives in the United States. In males, the death rate per 1,000 resident population was 10.4, and for females 1.1. A big breakthrough came in 1996, with the introduction of combination antiretroviral therapy for the disease. While there were around 39,000 deaths from HIV in the U.S. in 2022, the death rate had declined by 83 percent, resulting in HIV now being considered more as a chronic illness and not a death sentence.

On May 28, 1988, I was awarded my medical degree. Aside from the hooding ceremony, what I most recall was the recitation by graduates of the Hippocratic Oath, which includes: "I swear to fulfill, to the best of my ability and judgment, this covenant. I will respect the hard-won scientific gains of those physicians in whose steps I walk, and gladly share such knowledge as is mine with those who are to follow."

So, my dream of becoming a physician was finally realized at age 32. I embarked on a year-long rotating internship, which would be followed by three years of a residency in internal medicine at Faulkner Hospital in Boston.

In the summer of 1988, Kathy and I and the two boys moved to a rental house in Medfield, Massachusetts. Being a medical resident required that I worked around 80 hours a week, so Kathy was a stay at home mom. Our third child, Kaylin, was born on Sept. 14, 1991. She came out a roaring lioness. Over the years, she could turn the house upside down in an instant. (I often joked to people that if Kaylin had been our first child, she likely would have been an only child).

A year later, as our lease agreement was about to expire, Kathy and I set out to buy a house. We looked at several, but none were right. One day, our real estate agent called and told us she had a home in Medfield available for viewing later that day. Because of the short notice, we had no choice but to bring the three kids with us. The house had been built in 1750 and renovated in the 1930s and featured high ceilings and an open plan on the first floor. It sat on two acres abutting a pond. An in-ground swimming pool was just beyond an open small patio behind the house.

Kathy went from room to room, thinking how she could transform this house—which she said had "great character"—into something that would work for us. The boys were absolutely delighted with it, particularly the big yard and the pool. We bought it with our hearts and stored up many great memories during our 11 years there.

During those years, I was in private practice as an internist. Three years after we bought the house, Kathy took a job as a physical therapist at the Miriam Hospital in Providence.

In the mid-1990s, many health plans introduced the "managed care" insurance model (which, after several years, got dismantled due to backlash from patients and healthcare providers). In response, hospitals and physicians started organizing and merging into systems. In 1996, I was involved in assembling and leading a large independent primary care physician network in eastern Massachusetts. After nine years, it partnered with Tufts Medical Center, in Boston, to form the New England Quality Care Alliance. I served as the Alliance's inaugural board chairman for four years, during which time I remained active in my clinical practice.

Our youngest son, Brendan, arrived on Feb. 28, 1999, seven and a half years after Kaylin. Kathy called him "her 40th birthday present." As he grew, Brendan's demeanor recalled Patrick's—calm and thoughtful.

Of my four children, Brendan's influence on me was greater than that of his older siblings. Daniel, Patrick and Kaylin were born while I was in medical school and residency. During their early years, my studies, long shifts, on-call schedules, and occasional moonlighting shifts sharply limited how much meaningful time I could spend with them. I was well past all of that when Brendan arrived, so I enjoyed considerably more time with his infancy and toddler stages. Kathy wryly told her friends that Brendan was "my fourth, but George's first" child.

From birth, Dan and Patrick were very different. Dan was of medium build and height, had blond hair and brilliant blue eyes and was a righty. He was an active and coordinated child, but not much of a talker. In contrast, Patrick was tall, had dark hair, hazel eyes, and was left-handed. As an infant, he was rather sedentary. When toys rolled past him, he tended to just watch. As a joke, we occasionally called our second son "the slug."

The differing temperaments of our first two sons became more noticeable as the years rolled on. Dan was intense and focused but saw things in shades of gray. Patrick tended to view things in a binary manner, either black or white. As a strong Little League pitcher, Patrick had a very precise sense of the strike zone. When a pitch that Patrick knew was a strike was called a ball, his expression, although never disrespectful, clearly displayed his irritation. More than one umpire told me that my son's expressions weren't appreciated. I refrained from advising them to call pitches more accurately.

The boys also differed in their school performances. Both started in the Medfield system, which was consistently ranked among the top 10 in the state. At the time, the average class size was about 25 students. Dan was neither assertive nor troublesome in class, and, as he rarely asked questions, he became essentially invisible to the teachers. Patrick, on the other hand, was engaged and didn't hesitate to ask questions. One time, when more than half his class failed an important mathematics exam, he challenged the teacher on the fairness of the test questions. Kathy and I got a phone call about that.

We decided that Dan needed to be in a school with smaller classes. Despite his protests, we enrolled him in the seventh grade at St. Sebastian's School, an all-boys Catholic school in the nearby town of Needham. After a rather rocky start, it all came together for Dan. During his two years there, he thrived academically and athletically. He then transferred to Thayer Academy, a non-sectarian private school in Braintree, where Patrick joined him two years later. During winters, Dan played goalie on the varsity hockey team while Patrick played on the varsity basketball team. In the spring, they played together on the varsity lacrosse team. Seeing the brothers playing together brought us great joy.

Kaylin chose to remain in the town school system, where she did well academically, athletically and socially. As a child, Brendan happily attended many of his siblings' games, and the teammates of Patrick, Dan and Kaylin grew fond of this eager young fan. The three Beauregard boys became known to friends by their linked nicknames—Dbo, Pbo, and now Bbo. A highlight for Bbo came in February 2003 during the post-game celebration of a key victory by the Thayer hockey team. Knowing that Brendan's fourth birthday was just a few days away, the team presented him with a cake and gifts and sang happy birthday. Brendan beamed. Kathy and I watched with great pride and gratitude. Patrick relished the event. I think he already knew that he and his younger brother would become very close.

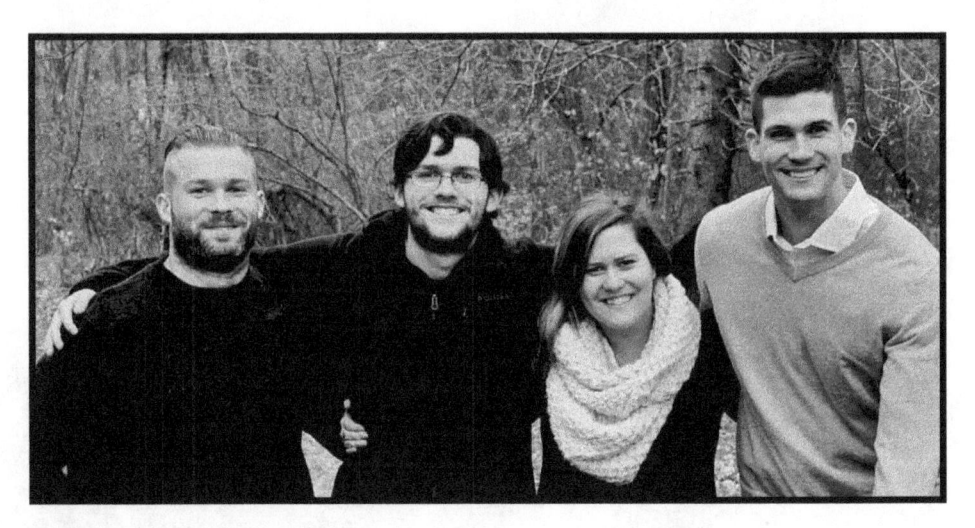

Photo Credit: Kim Neidermire

Through the teenage years of our first three children. Kathy and I attended weekly Mass with them. They all studied the Catechism and went through the sacrament of Confirmation, at around age 13. I largely kept the thought to myself, but, as a physician, I often saw bad things happen to good people and it occurred to me that God could be indifferent to the plight of individuals. When news surfaced in 2002 that the Archdiocese of Boston had covered up a clergy sex-abuse scandal involving 250 priests, attendance by Kathy and me at weekly Mass waned—and then ended.

It wouldn't be the last time that hard facts got in the way of faith.

# 5

# The Doctor

TOWARD THE END of my residency, I aspired to do a fellowship in either cardiology or hematology/oncology. Cardiology was appealing because at its basic level, the heart is just about two things—hydraulics and electricity. At an intimate level, it's about much more. For millennia, many civilizations viewed the heart the way the brain is understood today—the organ in which emotions and intelligence reside.

Hematology/oncology—blood and cancer medicine—includes the study of cells from the human embryo and bone marrow. The embryo and bone marrow produce stem cells and other substances, which in turn produce all the cells and tissues in the body. Sometimes, changes in cellular DNA cause mutations that result in the cell going rogue and wreaking havoc in the body. Hematology/oncology is a specialty in which you see a lot of people die.

But I had spent the previous eight years pursuing my dream of becoming a doctor. Kathy had shouldered a huge burden, and we were blessed with two fine sons and a daughter by then. I decided to defer applying for a fellowship and instead go into private practice in internal medicine—a specialty wherein physicians apply scientific knowledge and clinical expertise to diagnose and treat mostly adult patients presenting with a wide range of issues.

I was a solo practitioner for most of the following years. That meant seeing many thousands of patients and making countless decisions and diagnoses. I believe that science and a kind of art each play roles as doctors try to construct a diagnosis. There's nuance in this, and it takes varying lengths of time before you know whether you got it right. Your patients—and their families—pay the price if you're wrong.

Although a quixotic concept of the way doctors think exists, tremendous variation occurs at the individual physician level.

Most physicians making a diagnosis use a structured thinking process. It often starts with what's known as a diagnostic sieve—a mnemonic device in which each letter represents the cause of a medical condition. In diagnosing the patient, the doctor uses the mnemonic as a memory aid, running through each letter to reduce the likelihood that a particular condition is overlooked. For example, a common mnemonic is VITAMINCDE (vascular, infectious/inflammatory, traumatic/toxic, autoimmune/allergy, metabolic, iatrogenic/idiopathic, neoplastic, congenital, degenerative/drug-related, endocrine/exocrine). So-called illness scripts—mental summaries used to organize important information about a specific disease, including its causes, symptoms, diagnosis, and treatment—which occupy physician memories, play a role as well.

Within those conditions lie what are known as diagnostic imperatives—the "can't miss" diagnoses. These are disease states that, if not diagnosed, lead rapidly to disability or death, but can be mitigated, reversed or cured if treated. Consider, for example, that toe pain and discoloration in a patient with diabetes could be early dry gangrene, or atypical chest pain that's emanating from an aortic dissection, or a headache could be coming from a brain tumor. It goes without saying that physicians need to be acutely alert to diagnostic imperatives.

Most internists deal with a range of ages—from younger adult patients with single-organ problems to frail older patients with multiple chronic conditions. Despite the aspiration to consistently rely on scientific, rational decision-making, other factors come into play when physicians make diagnostic decisions: pattern recognition, intuition, and experience. Those factors usually assist in making a diagnosis; sometimes, they mislead.

Errors are not uncommon in medicine. Lawsuits alleging physician malpractice are filed relatively often in the U.S., averaging about 85,000 a year. About 30 percent of those claims fall into the failure-to-diagnose category. In the very small percentage of medical-malpractice cases that go to trial, 80 percent end up in favor of the defendant health-care provider. Damages are usually reduced on those cases that the plaintiffs win.

For me, part of internal medicine's allure is its similarity to detective work. Among other things, I used thinking tools such as Occam's razor or Hickam's dictum to fashion a diagnosis. Occam's razor suggests that the simplest explanation of a condition is the most likely to be accurate. (It's typically associated with the aphorism "When you hear hoofbeats, think horses, not zebras.") In medicine, that implies that diagnosticians should assume a single cause for multiple symptoms. On the other hand, one form of Hickam's dictum states: "A man can have as many diseases as he damn well pleases."

In practice, at times, I found maneuvering between these two opposites could be quite a challenge. When faced with an ill patient with multiple symptoms, I occasionally felt that I needed to hone in on a single one as the explanation for what was happening. But human bodies don't read medical textbooks, so the risk exists of not considering additional simultaneous diseases. With experience, when confronted with a patient with multiple complex symptoms, I started suspecting (and at times, expecting) that more than one disease was playing a role.

Regardless of what doctors think, studies show that patients remember only 49 percent of the information provided during conversations with doctors—and they think differently. In general, they are loss averse, often choosing not to act on a progressing illness that, if untreated, will result in greater harm in the future. (People with uncontrolled diabetes refusing to take insulin is an all too common occurrence). Said differently, most patients prefer certainty—"I'm fine how I am"—over the probability that an intervention would result in an improved future outcome. So, incorporating probability statistics in speaking to patients while blending scientific information with empathy and understanding can be challenging on many fronts.

But some doctors have therapeutic inertia too—for example, failing to make timely adjustments to therapies when treatment goals aren't met or not following evidence-based guidelines for the use of specific drugs at target doses. Despite strong evidence on mortality reduction, it's known that only 20 percent of patients with a particular type of heart failure are prescribed the most optimal therapy.

As the age, frailty and comorbidities—multiple ailments—of America's population increases, so do the number of disease-fighting weapons, such as diagnostic tools, novel drug therapies and new medical devices. Recently, computer-based, algorithmic clinical-decision-support-systems have been developed. Medical experts are expanding the use of artificial intelligence (AI) machine learning, and large language models like ClinicalKey AI to extract knowledge from data. This, of course, adds complexity to modern medicine.

Still, at the heart of being a doctor is the primacy of the physician-patient relationship. Over many years, I was a clinical instructor in internal medicine for students at the Tufts University School of Medicine, and I frequently had medical students rotate through my office. The first thing I told them was that being a doctor should be considered a privilege, one that needs to be taken absolutely seriously. The intimacy that a doctor earns from patients is virtually unparalleled among the professions. Patient visits are times of connection, and they should be held sacred. The strength of a good doctor depends heavily on his or her combination of intellectual/scientific rigor and compassion.

Many, probably most, patients come in feeling ill—and worried. (We worry a lot about many things). They may not know why they feel bad. The doctor is there to figure that out and advise an action. Sometimes, it's about more than just telling the patient to do something. So, a doctor's conscious decision-making occasionally includes helping the patient prioritize their consciousness of disease and misery, particularly when it's about that individual's real risk of a disease or a less than desirable outcome.

Patients reveal things to you that are extremely private: their family and social histories, tobacco and alcohol habits, sexual activity, mental health, living conditions, finances, and so on. Patient-physician conversations become the grist for decision making.

Good physicians listen intently to try to figure out what's going on. In his book *How Doctors Think*, Dr. Jerome Groopman points out that a doctor's decision-making process is susceptible to cognitive biases. The doctor may unknowingly rely on stereotypes, preconceived notions or heuristics—mental shortcuts—when diagnosing and treating patients. In that context, patient narratives and insights can provide valuable clues that might be otherwise overlooked. I recall hearing the adage, "If you listen long enough, the patient will tell you the diagnosis." (Of course, listening only adds value if the doctor is a good listener, which often isn't the case. A study published in the *Journal of General Internal Medicine* in 2019 found that the median time before a speaking patient was interrupted was just 11 seconds).

Having a trusted doctor who listens to your problems with some curiosity and who discusses with you what to do about them creates one of the more profound human relationships. The need to keep that information confidential is imperative. Patients, if they are fortunate, think of their primary care physicians as sympathetic confidantes with whom they feel a warm rapport.

The questions raised by patients can often be complicated and the answers can range from "you're fine" to "you're dying." It's almost always somewhere in between, but the answer can be life-changing, for good or bad. Doctors speak from a position of authority, so what we say—and how we say it—resonates with our patients in a manner that's quite different from advice provided by an auto mechanic.

As an internist, I prided myself on not being a doctor who reflexively referred patients with certain ailments immediately to specialists: for example, sending a patient with high blood sugar to an endocrinologist, or someone with knee pain to an orthopedist, or someone with a stomach ache to a gastroenterologist. I often told people that I didn't go through eight years of medical education without learning something, so, before referring to a specialist, I would order appropriate testing and evaluate the results. That way, I could establish a working diagnosis and valuable information to assist the specialist in taking the case forward. I couldn't do some tests, such as lung or bone marrow biopsies or cardiac catheterizations, so I had to leave that to the specialists. But before the consultation with the specialist, I would discuss with the patient the need for a work-up, and they usually appreciated the intent to make the impending visit more effective and efficient. It also provided me with the opportunity to hear what values and preferences my patient had about potentially facing a serious illness. And it let them know I was going to remain involved with their care going forward. They often felt reassured by that.

Over the years, I dealt with many patients who presented with new symptoms and signs that suggested a serious illness. Occasionally, my preliminary testing revealed the cause of their condition. Sometimes that meant I had to deliver catastrophic findings. I always tried to be candid, and yet not crush hopes. For example, I might say, "I have unfortunate news. All the test results indicate that you have an advanced-stage cancer, one with a low likelihood of surviving past five years at best. Of course, survival rates are based on broad populations, and might tell us little about how your individual situation will develop. What's more, advances in treatment might occur in the upcoming years, and if they do and are available, we can explore pursuing that as part of a clinical trial."

In speaking with an oncologist for the first time, many patients don't understand what they're hearing or can't recall it, as they have moved into anxiety, fear and fatalism. So, after a difficult consultation, I would help the patient review the results. I would speak about the treatment options that were available to prolong survival for an uncertain period and the likely side-effects and extreme discomfort associated with many therapies. When clinically appropriate, I'd also discuss the alternatives—palliative or hospice care—which most specialists don't do, given their unfamiliarity with the patient and family. I'd add, "I'm willing to discuss this with you anytime, but there is some urgency to acting sooner instead of later, and in the end, it's your choice of what you want to do. I'm not giving up on you, but from our time together over the years, I know quality of life is important to you. We're going to do everything we can to keep you comfortable and honor any special wishes you may have."

On numerous occasions throughout my clinical career, I said these words to people facing a terminal illness. (Regretfully, at times it felt like a recital).

In almost every instance, the patient and his/her family were devastated, but they eventually accepted the news and came around to making an appropriate decision, either to fight the disease through treatment, seek non-traditional alternative therapies, or settle for palliative care.

I recall one patient, the spouse of someone I knew. He was in his mid-50s and had a long history of avoiding medical care, but after many months of not feeling well, he acquiesced to seeing me. On the day I saw him, the lab called. His white blood cell count was greater than 50,000, the highest I'd ever seen (normal rarely goes beyond 10,000). Bypassing the emergency room, I directly admitted him to the hospital, where an expedited evaluation revealed he had acute promyelocytic leukemia. His condition was resistant to chemotherapy, so I spoke to him about the option of hospice care, which he accepted. "I don't want to die in a hospital," he said.

Bear in mind that a primary care physician might have to care for as many as 5,000 patients! That not only puts a strain on the time that can be spent with patients, but it puts a hard demand on the doctor's work/private-life balance. Thus, I should note that a paradox exists in the physician-patient relationship: Physicians should be very empathetic and yet remain detached.

I have felt the need over the years to compartmentalize my work life and my personal life. But many of my personal acquaintances (including close friends) elected to become my patients. Many assumed that Kathy would know about their conditions, though, of course, I never disclosed information about my patients to her.

A doctor can sometimes feel that he or she is on call all the time. Family members and others—sometimes complete strangers—rarely hesitate to say, "You're a doctor, can I ask you a medical question?" I almost always answer by saying that I would need to know more details before I could offer an opinion, adding, "You should consult your doctor."

For the most part, Kathy and my children tried to refrain from asking me questions about their various aches and pains. But they usually didn't have to because I was hypervigilant about their physical well-being. On a couple of occasions at home, I sutured wounds of my kids or their friends. I gave flu shots at home to Kathy and the kids. Kaylin always took delight in seeing five syringes prefilled with the flu vaccine in a Ziplock bag lying on the top shelf of our refrigerator. Kathy wasn't thrilled, but she liked the convenience of getting the shot at home. I also kept a small sharps container—a hard plastic box that is used to safely dispose of hypodermic needles. It was my version of home health.

But I didn't overreact to what I knew were low-acuity signs and symptoms. Good doctors can sense when people are really sick, whether or not they're stoic or dramatic. Occasionally, upon seeing a small cut, abrasion or wound that didn't require stitches, I would say, somewhat amusingly,

"All bleeding eventually stops." On two occasions, both Dan and Patrick witnessed with amazement as I left the viewing stands during a game and popped a dislocated shoulder of one their teammates back into the joint.

Perhaps because they saw the demands imposed on Kathy and me by our respective professions, none of our children pursued careers in health care. That was fine with us. They had to chart their own courses.

# 6

# Role Reversal

EARLY ONE WEEKDAY morning in September 2005, I got out of bed and took my usual pee in the bathroom off the master bedroom. I noticed what appeared to be a single bright red drop hitting the toilet water. As it sank, its red hue slowly twisted and dissipated like smoke from a lit candle. In seconds, it was gone. There was no discomfort or pain. The drops that followed were the customary clear yellow.

I wondered: Did I just pee a drop of blood? Or did I just imagine it?

I stood for a moment, staring into the white porcelain bowl while wishing I had a rewind button. Memories from medical school lectures, my residency and my practice flashed through my mind like a ticker tape. *Painless hematuria (blood in the urine) signifies cancer until proven otherwise.*

A few weeks earlier, I'd had some intermittent but significant right-side lower-back pain for a few days. It went away, and then periodically recurred. Remembering that, I wondered if perhaps the pain's cause was a kidney stone that had passed, and thus caused the hematuria—the blood in the urine. I dismissed that thought, as well as darker ones. For the next day or so, my urine was normal.

To my dismay, the blood reappeared several days later. This time, it was more than one drop. Again, there was no pain. I thought, or hoped maybe, that perhaps a small stone had lodged in my right ureter, the duct by which urine passes from the kidney to the bladder.

Again, I dismissed any concerns. After all, I was 49 and didn't have what are considered risk factors for kidney or bladder cancer: smoking, obesity, advanced age, high blood pressure, and workplace exposures (especially to cadmium, trichloroethylene or herbicides). A family history of kidney cancer is also considered a risk factor. I had to answer "unknown" on that question. But did I have a grim genealogy? What was perhaps significant, however, was that both of my adoptive parents had developed different types of urogenital cancer. That led me to speculate that environmental factors related to materials in our house and/or the land it sat on or around it had perhaps played a role.

When the bleeding appeared, I had probably applied the diagnostic sieve and considered the diagnostic imperatives on thousands of patients. Yet, I foolishly dismissed using them on myself. Like many other people whose job was patient care, I thought: patients get cancer, not doctors.

Although it did not occur daily, the frequency of my hematuria steadily increased, though it remained painless. I found myself having to get up several times during the night to urgently urinate. I did my best not to wake Kathy. As days went on, yellow and clear urine became yellow and clear with lots of red drops. The back pain returned on and off but wasn't always associated with the bleeding. Because I didn't want to alarm Kathy—then my wife of 23 years—and our four children, I decided to keep all this to myself for the time being. After this continued for a few weeks, and my urine started to look like cranberry juice, I finally realized that I had to have myself evaluated.

I would never advise any patient who described having symptoms like mine to take a wait-and-see approach. My avoidance of reality came from fear of finding out what was wrong. If the news were bad, what would it mean for Kathy and our children?

At the time, Dan was a freshman at Connecticut College. Patrick was in his junior year at Thayer Academy. Kaylin was in the eighth grade, and Brendan, at six, was a first grader. I was in private practice and Kathy was the family's full-time domestic engineer. As a family, we were thriving. Life lessons of parents and children were shared.

The year before, we had built a new home on a quiet street in a different part of Medfield. Kathy and I had enjoyed contributing to the interior and exterior design of the two-story colonial, which featured an open floor plan, four bedrooms, a wraparound porch and sat on a little less than an acre of land. My father, having built the house I grew up in, did frequent walk throughs and commented on the quality of the craftsmanship and the sturdiness of the construction. We moved in during November 2004.

November 1, 2005, found me supine on a clinic bed in a free-standing imaging center undergoing an abdominal and pelvic ultrasound. As a former X-ray technologist, I had some familiarity with how a normal bladder would appear on ultrasound. What I saw in the grainy images captured by the transducer wasn't a normal-looking bladder. The right ureter was enlarged. More notable was what looked like a golf-ball sized soft tissue density at the base of my bladder. Knowing that I was a physician, the technician pointed it out, saying, "Do you see that? I don't know what it is, but there's a mass there." He promised a radiologist's report within 24 hours.

A day or so later, the official interpretation came. It read in part, "a soft tissue density is seen in the base of the bladder toward the right. While this could represent thrombus, I cannot rule out a primary mucosal lesion. The lesion measures approximately 4 X 5 cm in diameter."

In other words, this didn't look like a blood clot. I thought: *You've probably got cancer.* Fuck.

I took a deep breath and swallowed hard. How the hell would I tell Kathy and the kids? What will this mean for me and, more importantly, them?

I called Paul C, a trusted urologist colleague. He said he would see me the next day and perform a cystoscopy (a procedure that in men involves the insertion of a fiber optic scope though the penis into the bladder, allowing its direct visualization). He could do it in his office and told me to come in around 4:30 in the afternoon.

That evening, Brendan and Marley, our Bichon Frise, greeted me when I came home. The night before, Brendan and I had spent a happy Halloween as I took him around in his Batman costume. I found Kathy in the same upstairs bathroom where my first signs of cancer had appeared. She was doing something with her hair. Early in our relationship, I became aware that Kathy's intuition was uncannily strong—and almost always accurate. Upon seeing me, a worried look descended over her face like a window shade being pulled down. "Is there something wrong?" she asked.

"I have something to tell you. You might want to sit down."

As if invisible hands were pushing down on her shoulders, she sat on the edge of the hot tub. For me, words that previously had the structure of unburnt logs in a fireplace had become ashes. I did my best to spit them out, explaining events in as coherent and reassuring a way as I could manage.

Even if it is cancer, I told her, "I'm sure everything will be fine. I'll understand if you're really upset with me for not letting you know sooner, but the truth is, I didn't want to worry you. I was scared, too. I have an appointment tomorrow with a good urologist I know."

Kathy calmly processed the alarming and unexpected news. After taking a deep breath, she said, "Well, I'm obviously surprised and concerned to hear this. At least for now, it's the only information you have. There's more to be done and to learn. We'll take it one step at a time. I'm sorry that you've had to go through this. I'll be right by your side."

To say the least, our interactions during the rest of the night were a bit awkward and subdued, with each of us trying to think of how we would navigate the possible scenarios ahead. We both slept poorly.

The following day started with rounds on hospitalized patients of mine, then a full schedule of seeing patients in the office. As someone with strong compartmentalization skills, I made it through the day without failing my patients.

Late that afternoon, I headed back to where my day had started—Faulkner Hospital, where Dr. C had his office. Kathy accompanied me. Over the years, I referred many patients to Dr. C. The feedback from these patients was nearly always positive. He was a consummate professional.

When he met us in the empty waiting room, his expression subtly displayed concern. He had seen the ultrasound report. He escorted me to an exam room, where his nurse was waiting. Kathy stayed alone in the waiting room. I donned the depressing disposable pale blue hospital gown and sat on the exam table, waiting with apprehension. Paul explained, "We'll start by having you lie down and injecting lidocaine into your penis to numb things up." The pain from that was fleeting. And away we went.

After completing the cystoscopy, Paul left the room and went back to the waiting room. I walked a few feet down the hallway to the first restroom I could find. I started to urinate a forceful stream. The pain was excruciating, as if I were peeing shards of glass. Slight relief finally came when I finished. Whew! That really fucking hurt!

Being a physician often involves interpreting symptoms and feelings expressed by patients. Well, now I know what having a cystoscopy feels like.

When I returned to the waiting room, I sensed that Paul was struggling to keep his composure. I braced myself. "As you know, you have a mass in your bladder," he told Kathy and me. "I got a very good view of it. It's pretty angry looking, so I suspect it's not benign. I tried to remove as much as I could. It would've been pretty risky to scrape deeper and risk puncturing your bladder. I know I didn't get all of it." He said I would need a transurethral resection of a bladder tumor—bladder surgery. I thanked him for seeing me so quickly. As Kathy and I left, I began thinking about the long and very difficult days to come.

I also thought about whether I had experienced early warning signs, before the blood in my urine. The year before, I had started having episodic palpitations—irregular, often rapid, heartbeats—a condition known as paroxysmal atrial fibrillation. I conferred with a cardiologist and tests found no structural abnormalities of my heart. I later discovered that studies suggested an association between atrial fibrillation and certain cancers, including bladder cancer.

And I remembered again that both my adoptive parents had developed different types of urogenital cancer.

At home that evening, Kathy and I spoke with Patrick, 17, and Kaylin, 14. Their reactions were very different. Pat listened carefully and remained calm. "Everything will be fine, Dad," he assured me. Kaylin, looking horrified, immediately started crying. Although she didn't say it then, she wanted to ask me if I was going to die. Sleep eluded me that night.

Dan, 19, was at Connecticut College, in New London, Connecticut, where he had been recruited to play ice hockey. I didn't want to relay the news over the phone, so I called and asked if Kathy and I could come down and take him out for dinner. He was delighted.

We drove to New London and took him to a nearby Olive Garden. Following some casual conversation, we revealed the bad news. We asked that he stay positive and continue his education and hockey in the strongest way possible. He sat stoically and said he understood and would await further information. The drive home from New London seemed to take longer than usual. I worried that Dan's college experience was going to be much more difficult going forward.

As Brendan was only six, Kathy and I felt that he couldn't understand what cancer meant and therefore needed to be shielded from this bad news. Some of our close friends advised us similarly. Accordingly, we talked about Daddy having to go see some doctors for some troubles he was having. There was no mention of the Big C to him. Brendan later told us he recently had been having dreams about bad people attacking our family. He likened it to *Star Wars*: Darth Vader and the Imperial Army against the Jedi and the Rebel Alliance. He brought out his *Star Wars* figurines and demonstrated a battle to us. He said the Alliance would win.

We generally demanded very few but important things from our children. First and foremost, we asked them to be respectful, courteous and kind. We wanted them to stick up for their siblings and help others who couldn't defend themselves. In school, effort mattered more than grades. We could provide tutoring if necessary. In athletics, we reminded them that they were part of a team, and if they scored a goal or touchdown or hit a home run, they should act as if they'd done it before. Each knew that any grandstanding would result in me walking onto the field and escorting them off.

With my cancer, Kathy and I told the kids that while this preliminary news wasn't good, I needed additional evaluations and testing to determine the extent of the disease. Once known, that would provide information—and perhaps choice—on the best treatment options. Their job will be to continue what they've been doing in the best manner they can. In school, on the playing field or at home, they were to stay steady at the wheel. We're all in this together. We will not let cancer rule us.

Bad as my situation was, worse was to come.

Having done my internal medicine residency at Faulkner Hospital and having been on the active medical staff there for some 15 years, I knew many of the hospital's clinical and support services staff. On November 7, as I progressed through the protocols of the pre-op area, some of my interactions with the staff I knew were awkward, but more often comforting. Eventually, I lay on an operating room table, my consciousness surrendering to anesthesia. Dr. C performed the surgery, which was relatively simple. About an hour later, I ascended from the depths of complete sedation. Kathy drove me home.

As a previously healthy 49-year-old, I didn't resemble the typical bladder cancer patient. The average age of people diagnosed with the disease then was 73. I had none of the known risk factors. A few days later, Dr. C called. The pathology results didn't look good. There was evidence that the cancer had penetrated the bladder wall and invaded the deeper muscular layer beneath it, known as muscle-invasive bladder cancer (MIBC). I would have to undergo major surgery.

Before treatment begins for any patient with cancer, doctors need to know how much cancer exists, and where it is. The globally accepted method for organizing that information is the TNM (tumor, node and metastasis) system, which provides a standardized method for classifying the anatomic extent (local, regional and distant) of the disease. Accordingly, TMN reflects the prognosis.

Though assigning a stage to a case of cancer started over a hundred years ago, it has since undergone many iterations. In 1982, a single TNM classification comprising staging algorithms for almost all cancers emerged and remains in use.

To determine the stage of my cancer, I underwent CT scans of my abdomen and lungs. Fortunately, the images did not reveal distant spread. However, the pathology report of the tumor specimens demonstrated a poorly differentiated cancer type with local lymphovascular invasion, raising the specter of micro metastasis (small numbers of cancer cells that have spread from the primary tumor to other parts of the body and are too few and small to be detected by a diagnostic test). Poorly differentiated cancer cells behave more aggressively than well differentiated ones, which portends a worse outcome. At best, my stage was T2bNXMO. In layman terms, that would be stage 2 bladder cancer. The presence of lymphovascular invasion—providing a pathway to other destinations—suggested that I probably had at least stage 3 disease, not good.

I was now a patient with cancer. Transitional cell carcinoma is a slow-developing cancer with a latency period—the amount of time from exposure to a toxin or disease-causing agent—of anywhere up to 15 years and the manifestation of symptoms. So, I didn't think that my irresponsible reluctance to be evaluated sooner had resulted in my having this more advanced stage.

Still, being told *you have cancer* is a life-changing experience. Not only does it inflict trauma, it also assaults your preconceived notions and plans. Any likelihood of having a care-free everyday existence gets erased. You worry about the future while trying to live in the moment. It's as if you've become a manifestation of Albert Einstein's theory of wave particle duality—light behaves as both a wave and as a particle. As he wrote: "We have two contradictory pictures of reality; separately neither of them fully explains the phenomena..., but together they do." Kathy described the experience as being in purgatory.

Most people who receive a cancer diagnosis want to know one thing above all else: their prognosis. "How much time do I have left?" Even though I knew my situation was an anomaly, I found myself wanting to know the number.

At the time I was diagnosed, people with cancers that extended through the bladder to the surrounding tissue or had spread to nearby lymph nodes or organs had a five-year survival rate of about 43 percent. Lucky me, I thought. I might actually live to see my 55th birthday. I'd just crossed over into the Twilight Zone. Nonetheless, I couldn't imagine my life without futurity beyond five years.

Over my years in practice, I had had many discussions about survival rates with patients who had newly diagnosed cancers. I would remind them that statistics are drawn from broad populations, so applying them to individual cases can be misleading. What's more, in clinical studies, life expectancy is typically measured and reported as five-year survival rates and mortality. On the surface, those rates are easy to compute, but there are subtle distinctions in interpreting them. Furthermore, they're based on the exact treatments used during the study period.

In my case, I clearly wasn't like the (older) study populations, and no granular data about my age band existed. So now I had to give myself the same caveats and comforts that I'd been offering patients for years.

As this experience unfolded, a recurring thought ran through my mind: Better that it's happening to me than to Kathy or one of the kids.

I explained my situation to immediate and extended family members and close friends. The reactions varied, ranging from hysterical to rational and supportive. Kathy and I vowed that we would work to remain positive—and we wanted others to try to do so as well. Whether we liked it or not, we were on a non-stop train ride from which we couldn't disembark until the ordeal was over. Our mantra became, "Either get on the train and stay in the light or get off."

Several weeks later, family members and friends were wearing blue rubber wristbands with two words: "GEO FORCE."

Living in the Boston area for most of my life, I knew that many bladder cancer specialists were available, and so I rapidly assembled a list. First, I saw three surgeons, associated with three different hospitals.

The first described in a slow, deliberate manner the various aspects of the major surgery I needed. In medical terminology, it was called a "radical cystectomy, small bowel resection and construction of an orthotopic ileal neobladder." In everyday language, it meant the complete removal of my bladder and nearby lymph nodes. Then the surgeon would create an internal pouch derived from part of my small intestine that would serve as my replacement bladder, called a neobladder. (Over time, a neobladder expands and holds an amount of urine similar to a natural bladder). Given the location of my cancer and the chance that some of it may have spread to my prostate gland, the surgeon advised complete removal of that as well.

At the least, he said, doing all the above would require "about a five-hour operation. You'll need to be in the hospital for somewhere between one and two weeks." Post-discharge, I would have an indwelling Foley catheter (a flexible tube inserted through the penis and into the bladder to drain urine), a suprapubic catheter (inserted into the bladder through a cut through the lower abdomen) and various other tubes and drains in place for as long as six weeks.

The muscles of the small intestine and urinary bladder are different, but they are both considered to be primarily involuntary. Their contractions, controlled by our autonomic nervous system, are independent of voluntary nerve activity. Accordingly, the surgeon said that I would need to "train" my neobladder to avoid inadvertently peeing myself. That training involved doing Kegel exercises—typically recommended for strengthening pelvic muscles in women with urinary stress incontinence. I would also need to urinate frequently, probably at least every four hours. Performing the exercises multiple times a day would result in my neobladder developing some pseudo-voluntary muscle control.

Removing the prostate gland usually leaves the patient with some permanent erectile dysfunction. The current surgical procedure incorporates a nerve-sparing technique that avoids cutting adjacent nerves. Although this technique increases the chance of retaining near-normal sexual and urinary function, I would likely still be left with some permanent erectile dysfunction and incontinence.

Talk about feeling as if you're going to resemble a much older man overnight!

The surgeon recounted the facts in a monotone, sitting with his arms folded, resting atop his office desk. At one point during his lengthy description, I felt as if I were starting to float above my body, like a balloon that had lost its tether, looking down on myself and Kathy. For the first time ever, I felt that I was having an out-of-body experience.

The last surgeon I consulted was John L, who was at a large hospital northwest of Boston, and was highly recommended by a trusted colleague. The first thing that Dr. L told me when he entered the exam room brought comfort. "I know how you're feeling today," he said. "A little over a year ago, I was the one sitting in that chair. I'd been diagnosed with kidney cancer and needed to have a kidney removed. I did what I had to do, recovered and here I am, doing what I love to do. Helping people. I've done what you need some 800 times now with very good outcomes. I'll give you my data if you want to see it." The icebreaking was accomplished.

Dr. L was tall, had a large frame, dark hair, striking brown eyes and a magnetic smile. His voice was a baritone with an Italian accent. I studied his hands. Robotic-assisted surgery for my condition was still in its early stages. In medical school I learned that hands are one of the body's most complex pieces of engineering, and I witnessed doctors using them with skill and dexterity. Dr. L's large hands were well groomed, with clean, smooth skin and fingers that were well-defined and showed well-toned muscles. These qualities suggested that he could easily manipulate small objects in the small spaces within the pelvic cavity with great precision.

Each of the three surgeons I consulted recommended the same type of operation. I decided to have Dr. L perform the surgery. It was an easy decision, given his extensive experience and bedside manner. Although Kathy said the choice of surgeon was mine to make, she felt the same way.

Chemotherapy options presented more difficult choices. Because of my cancer's aggressive nature—and the presence of local invasion—there was a high risk of it spreading to distant sites, if it already hadn't. I faced choices about the timing of the chemotherapy in relation to the surgery—before (neoadjuvant) or after (adjuvant)—as well as the type of chemotherapy (different drug regimens). Data available on outcomes were mixed. Again, I sought several opinions and consulted three respected oncologists, each from a different and renowned academic medical center in Boston.

One was a colleague of mine—Dr. John E, at Tufts New England Medical Center. Although Jack (as he was commonly called) specialized in breast cancer, I was confident that he would provide impressive advice and treatment. We met in a large waiting room next to the cancer center reception area. Kathy was meeting him for the first time. Jack and I started by talking about work-related things—our way of warming up to unpleasant matters. Kathy quickly interrupted. "Excuse me, I'm not here to talk about your work relationship. I'm here to find out if you can help my husband."

"Yes, I can help George get through this," he said calmly. He reached to the floor to pick up a stack of articles from medical journals and as carefully as one would place an infant, he laid them on his lap. "As you know, George doesn't fit the typical profile of people who develop bladder cancer. Since he reached out to me last week, I've been researching the most current evidence on chemotherapy for advanced stage disease. I've reached out to some other clinical researchers as well." He handed me the pile of articles. "Why don't you take these home, go through them, and we can discuss further when we meet next week."

Jack and the two other oncologists I saw each had different recommendations. Jack initially recommended a two-drug regimen that would be administered before the surgery. The second oncologist was affiliated with the renowned Dana-Farber Cancer Institute and had cared for several of my patients over the years. When I saw him he described my cancer as "like a wolf that has chewed its way out of a metal cage. It's out." He was implying the probability of micrometastasis. The grim ferocity of the simile set me back. I wondered: If my stage is actually higher, should I even consider undergoing treatments that will have a profound negative effect on my physical and mental health only to later discover that it was futile? Note to the doctor—and myself—find a different way to say that the cancer might not be confined to a single organ. Be honest, but don't extinguish the hope and the fight response that sometimes can improve outcomes.

This doctor recommended a four-drug regimen that could be administered in part before and then after the surgery. His preferred recommendation, however, was adjuvant chemotherapy. (Chemotherapy administered after the surgery). I also recall him saying something like "If you choose me as your medical oncologist, your life schedule belongs to me." Another rankling remark. Kathy's silent response to his statement: "You're [expletive deleted] out!"

After consulting with the oncologists, I had to choose: Which regimen would provide the highest probability of a five- or ten-year survival rate? Expert reviews of clinical trials that compared different chemotherapy regimens in younger patients with advanced bladder cancer did not exist. That aside, treatment decisions involve more considerations than evidence alone. They need to be individualized to the specific patient or situation—and to incorporate patients' preferences.

Relying on treatment protocols derived from clinical trials that perhaps included only a small number of people with early-onset bladder cancer essentially leads to a "one size fits all" approach. And ill-suited for an anomalous case like mine.

It felt as if my longevity depended on a dart toss or a spin of a roulette wheel. My choices were: (a) undergo the surgery first, recover from that, then undergo chemotherapy with its side-effects; (b) have the chemotherapy first, recover from that and then have the major surgery; (c) undergo two cycles of chemotherapy first, recover from that, then have the surgery, recover from that, and then have the third and fourth cycles of chemotherapy. Contemplating the varieties of this wash-rinse-repeat cycle was mind-bending and numbing.

Pick the most effective therapy and hope for the best outcome—meaning I'd probably be a 10-year survivor. Pick a lesser one and I was headed for the express check-out lane. What I did know, however, was that I needed to make a choice quickly—and never look back. While I knew there is no evidence that having a positive attitude improves the chance of survival, other studies show it leads to a better quality of life.

Within a few days, my brain and my gut made my choice. Per Jack's recommendation, I would undergo the chemotherapy first and then have the surgery.

The very word "chemotherapy" has an ominous sound, but in fact the treatment has an interesting history and has resulted in tremendous advances against certain cancers. Chemotherapy's early use, weirdly, began with the German introduction of chemical warfare during World War I. Scientists discovered that the weapon nitrogen mustard could effectively treat lymphoma-type cancers (though obviously it was devastating in other respects).

Shortly after World War II, Dr. Sidney Farber, a pediatric pathologist at Harvard Medical School who's considered the father of modern chemotherapy, successfully used close chemical relatives of the vitamin folic acid to induce remission in children with a certain acute leukemia. Initially, the results were met with ridicule from the medical establishment. But soon researchers also found success against cancer with platinum compounds, such as cisplatin and oxaliplatin—two very toxic but effective agents still in use. Today, there are more than 100 types of chemotherapy drugs. Different types are used to treat different cancers. In all, the discovery that certain toxic chemicals administered in combination could cure certain cancers ranks as one of the greatest discoveries in modern medicine.

Chemotherapy can kill cancerous cells through several mechanisms, but at its most basic, chemotherapy shuts down the wild and uncontrolled divisions and growth that occur in cancer cells. The major problem is that these drugs don't differentiate between healthy and cancerous cells. Healthy cells, whose growth typically slows under chemotherapy, usually recover, while cancer cells usually don't. Still, the side effects can be debilitating—among them, damaged reproductive hormones and fertility, affecting both sperm and eggs.

Chemotherapy can be either *systemic*, which means that drugs are sent through the bloodstream to reach cells throughout the body, or *regional*, when they are directed to a specific body part. My regimen would be systemic and consist of four cycles of the combination of Cisplatin (among the most powerful and toxic agents) and Gemcitabine. These treatments would be administered once monthly for four months.

Cisplatin works by interfering with the DNA in cancer cells and triggering cell stress responses. Once it enters the cancer cells, it bonds with the DNA strands—a process called DNA crosslinking—and distorts the DNA structure, preventing normal DNA replication. In addition, it temporarily stops elements of the process whereby the cell copies itself, thus promoting the eventual cell death.

Gemcitabine works by competing with the natural building blocks of DNA during the replication process. When incorporated into the growing DNA chain, the chain can't be extended, eventually shutting down DNA synthesis.

At that time, immunotherapy was gaining use as a treatment that harnessed the body's natural ability to attack cancer cells. Between his initial evaluation of my case and the follow-up visit, Jack had done more research. He discovered that my type of cancer contained a protein that promoted the growth of cancer cells. Adding an immunotherapy drug known as trastuzumab (brand name Herceptin), which blocks the ability of cancer cells to receive growth-promoting chemical signals, might enhance the chemotherapy's effectiveness. Jack advised adding it to my regimen. Given how deeply I trusted him and my willingness to throw everything at this disease, I went for it. The cost for a single dose of Herceptin at the time was $8,000 to $10,000. Knowing that I would require three treatments, I was relieved that my insurance would cover it in full.

On November 23, 2005, Kathy and I headed to the Tufts Medical Center Cancer Infusion Center in downtown Boston, where intravenous medications are delivered directly into the bloodstream. As we arrived, we noticed an elderly, somewhat frail-looking woman slowly walking toward us on the other side of the sunlit hallway. I quickly recognized her as Helen, a patient of mine for many years who was undergoing treatment for a blood cancer. I introduced her to Kathy. "It's so nice to meet you, my dear," Helen said. "The doctor always talks about you and your children with such joy and pride." She turned to me. "Doctor, are you here seeing patients? How nice."

I paused, briefly debating whether to explain, considering that Helen had more important things to deal with. "I'm sorry to report that I'm here as a patient today. I've been recently diagnosed with cancer."

She looked stunned and told me I was far too young and was needed by my patients. We hugged and I told her I would fight it. "People like you have inspired me over the years," I told her.

I checked into the center and was escorted to my chair, where I would sit while being infused. My nurse greeted me warmly and began asking the necessary questions and preparing the equipment. Oncology nurses are a special breed. Angels on Earth. I spent much of the day seated in a somewhat comfortable, tan-colored chair, intravenously receiving the first cycle of the two drug regimens. (Herceptin would be added to subsequent cycles).

I went home feeling pretty good. I understood that the side effects of chemotherapy are often cumulative. They would eventually declare themselves loud and clear. The next day was Thanksgiving, on which we usually hosted the feast. For most of our guests that day, the mood was as festive and joyful as usual. The turkey dinner was delicious. I ate well. I had been advised not to drink alcohol while undergoing chemotherapy. Nonetheless, I enjoyed a little Asti Spumante and a glass of wine. It all felt a bit surreal for Kathy and me, but we had already determined that we would do our best to live our lives as normally as possible—cancer would not dominate us.

The first side effects came about a week later. My early-morning routine had always included starting with a cup of coffee. But this time, the first sip tasted awful. I took another sip. Just as bad! Kathy was sitting in her usual chair, enjoying her first cup. "Did you buy a different type of coffee?" I asked. No. She said hers tasted normal.

I thought: And so, it began. By the end of the week, a metallic taste had taken temporary residence in my mouth. After that, I started losing my sense of taste and smell, until they were completely gone. It's very difficult to be hungry when whatever you're putting in your mouth tastes like cardboard. Eventually, I virtually stopped eating. Substantial weight loss followed.

Although I was expecting it, the hair-loss episode was particularly unnerving. One morning, while I was showering, the hair on my head started coming out in clumps. Over the next few days, the hair on my armpits, chest, pubic area and limbs followed suit. Weirdly however, I retained the mustache I had had since I was 18.

My extreme fatigue was quickly accompanied by living in a dissociative state most of the time. This was particularly unnerving to Kathy and my children. I think that even our dog, Marley, sensed something wasn't quite right. One day before the Christmas holidays, Kathy was wrapping gifts with her sisters. I sat motionless, staring into space in the same room. My mind seemed nearly void of coherent thought. Kathy told me later that seeing me like that was very disconcerting to her sisters.

One of the hardest things you learn going through cancer treatment is that you must relinquish routine activities that you used to do—such as cutting the grass, raking the leaves, going to the dump, etc.—and let other people handle the chores. In short order, one of my sister-in-laws asked for my credit card. Following that exchange, we had hired a landscaping company and a waste-removal service.

In late November of 2005, I took my first ever leave of absence from my clinical duties.

Shortly after my first round of chemotherapy, two of Kathy's friends organized a meal train for our family. Two or three nights a week, people, some of whom we didn't know, would bring their best dishes, leaving them on our front porch, with serving instructions and encouraging notes. Not having to cook dinner every night afforded some relief to Kathy. Our children thoroughly enjoyed the fine fare. Most nights, I hardly ate, because of nausea or simply because I couldn't taste the food.

The meal train lasted until I was completely recovered from my surgery and feeling better—a span of almost five months. Toward the end, Kathy reached out to one of the organizers, Mary Piccolo, and told her that it could stop. "It can't stop yet," Mary said. "There are still a lot of names on the list who haven't yet contributed their meal and they really want to. I know it's easier to give than receive, but you have to try to give yourself some grace to accept this. You need to let them do that." So the culinary delights kept coming. When they finally ended, Patrick joked, "Does this mean we have to eat just Mom's cooking again?" Kathy frowned. I tried to conceal my grin.

Deciding when to have my surgery was up to me. I had been advised to wait a few weeks after completing the chemotherapy, but not too long—after all, the wolf was out of the cage. One date offered was February 28, 2006, Brendan's seventh birthday. As much as I didn't want to disrupt his fun, part of me felt that having surgery that day would add positive karma.

With Kathy by my side, I arrived at the hospital at 6 a.m. My dad and Kathy's younger sisters, Colleen and Kara, accompanied us. Once I was settled into the pre-op holding area and the pre-op ritual was completed, Kathy was allowed in. We had a difficult "see you later and I love you" exchange, followed by a firm hand squeeze and a kiss. Then I was wheeled into the OR, given anesthesia, and Dr. L went to work.

The surgery took four-and-a-half hours. By around 3 p.m., I was in the recovery room. When you wake up after anesthesia, you're surprised that hours have gone by. I slowly ascended from the depths of that induced deep sleep (a great place to be for someone who hasn't slept well for several months) to a semi-awake state. I blinked, trying to focus on my surroundings. Blurrily, I saw people next to my bed, speaking to me softly. Kathy was firmly gripping my hand. Her love and energy seemed to run up my arm and course through my body. I fell back into an intermittent sleep.

A nurse told Kathy that only two people would be allowed to visit me at a time. Kathy had prepped Dan and Patrick on what to expect. I was covered up to my neck by a sheet and layers of blankets. Dan leaned over and hugged me, sobbing while saying, "You're going to be okay, Dad." Patrick stood at the foot of the bed and calmly, stoically assessed my situation while rubbing my feet. He, too, said, "You're going to be okay, Dad."

Around 2:30 the next morning, I was transferred to a private room upstairs. As the post-op protocol called for frequent checks of my vital signs, the nurses and their aides kept popping in and out in kind of a sleepless

Chinese water torture. But what I most remember about this private room was a big clock on the wall, with its large black minute and hour hands revolving slowly, while the smaller, red second hand tiptoed through the seconds. The otherwise quiet room seemed to amplify the clock's Tick Tock, Tick Tock. Because I couldn't move my body, I felt I was a prisoner of that clock. Under those conditions, time became everything and nothing.

I took my first glance under the covers to see what my abdomen looked like. While a large dressing covered most of it, I saw that many things were now sticking out of me. The incision ran from slightly below the end of my sternum and ended just above my pubic area. Several inches lateral to that incision, and on both sides, I had a tube to drain fluids from under the incision and another to handle urine. The central line—a large IV catheter used for giving fluids, medications and drawing blood—remained in my neck.

Most annoying was the nasogastric tube—a type of medical catheter inserted through the nose and into the stomach. Abdominal surgery typically results in a temporary reduction in intestinal activity, which can become life-threatening if prolonged. Nasogastric tubes are routinely inserted to mitigate that risk until the intestines become active. In me it frequently provoked my gag reflex.

All those tubes were just what was visible. Tucked inside was a Foley catheter—a flexible tube that is inserted into the bladder to drain urine—and nephrostomy tubes that provided an alternative pathway for urine to exit the body.

I closed my eyes and hoped that I could fall asleep. Tick Tock, Tick Tock.

Kaylin—14 at the time—visited me on post-op day four. Unfortunately, for her and for me, it was my worst day of recovery, and I looked it—pale, sweating, undergoing waves of nausea and vomiting. Kay was horrified and was quickly escorted out by an aunt.

I gradually improved enough to walk up and down the long hallway of the unit. Positioned in front of my rolling walker was my rolling IV pole, with clear plastic bags filled with intravenous fluids and at times vitamin supplements. For many days, it seemed to be my constant companion. My urinary catheter bag was also on the pole, displaying my sloshing yellow urine—embarrassing, even to a physician like me.

What I hated most, though, was the nasogastric tube. It would only come out when I resumed a basic bodily function—the ability to pass gas, indicating that my intestines had resumed functioning. My first post-op fart emerged late one evening. Excited, I summoned the surgical resident on call. He told me removal could wait until morning. I threatened to call Dr. L. He grudgingly removed the tube. The relief was immediate. Hallelujah! I've never celebrated flatulence so much,

On post-op day six, John L appeared wearing his long white coat over green scrubs. He looked at me with a big smile. "All of your pathology reports from the surgical specimens are back," he told me. "They're all clean. I believe you are cured. Of course, we're going to need to follow you with serial scans and check-ups for a while."

The elation I felt was tempered by the many years of seeing patients of mine who, having been "cured" of cancer, suffered relapses.

Along with all my attached appliances and accouterments, I was discharged to go home on March 8, 2006. I was ecstatic. Although a tough recovery lay ahead, I felt that the worst of this ordeal was behind me. That was true, but there was plenty of stuff to come.

I was hobbled and weak and tethered to my appliances. When I wasn't in bed, I sat in a recliner we'd moved to the second-floor bedroom, with tubes hanging over the armrests. Frequent check-ins by family members would lift my spirits. My loving, inexhaustible caregiver, Kathy, was omnipresent. My children came in and chatted or watched the large-screen television with me. Meals were brought up to me. I couldn't shower, so cleaning came from sponge baths. Slowly, I gained strength.

Nine days after my discharge, I returned to the hospital, and the various tubes were removed. That apparently set off an infection, and sepsis set in.

I was hospitalized again. I imagined the wall clock saying, "Welcome back! I've missed you!" I spent another 10 days in the hospital.

Within a couple of weeks of returning home from that second hospital stay, I surprised Kathy by booking a three-day getaway in June to The Reefs, a luxury resort in Bermuda. Our stay there was a great pleasure. Unable to swim, I enjoyed walking and lounging on the beach. I began to feel that I was returning to normality. I joyfully resumed my clinical practice in May 2006.

Throughout my cancer marathon and for the six months after, I took a frequent inventory of how my family was handling the situation. Kathy did everything she could to support me through my physical and psychological ordeal. She was unwavering in trying to keep us moving forward. Being a physical therapist with extensive experience in treating musculoskeletal and cardiopulmonary ailments and wound care, she performed many of the services that the visiting nurse would otherwise have done. I don't think that most spouses would have the willingness or skill to provide daily dressing changes that sometimes involved treating a partial separation of my abdominal incision. She never complained and tried to keep my spirits high.

Cancer and its treatments create a particularly harsh reality for young children and teenagers. While my kids had moments of sadness and anxiety, I'm proud to say they remained steady at the wheel as they went about their regular activities. Their experiences with my illness served as valuable life lessons for them.

When my treatment was finally over, nearly 10 months had passed from the first day I saw blood in my urine. Having come through it, I hoped our new normal would be realized and things would be fine. While that was true in our regular daily activities, our psyches were sometimes train wrecks. Having cancer is a non-linear experience; there are lots of mood swings. Because Kathy and I each thought, "It's only me thinking this way," we rarely shared our feelings.

For many years, she and I mostly behaved as people of science—rational, organized and not prone to act on impulse alone. Now we found ourselves wobbling and flailing. It was as if we had become human tops that were slowing down. Far from the life we had known before cancer, we were unsure about how to move forward. I remember telling Kathy that I didn't know whether to look up, down, east or west. She felt the same way. My clinical experience led me to recognize that we were probably both suffering from mild depression and post-traumatic stress disorder. We found ourselves arguing more than ever before, simple disputes often escalating into shouting. Admitting finally that we needed counseling wasn't easy, but at times vulnerabilities can become strengths.

We were given the name of a psychologist in the nearby town of Needham. Jocelyn Barrett, a woman in her mid-sixties, was charming and soft-spoken. She was an active outdoorswoman and particularly enjoyed kayaking.

The therapy proved valuable. On a weekly or biweekly basis—sometimes individually, other times together—Kathy and I went through the layers of physical and emotional stress of the past months. It was hard work. Through listening and questioning, Jocelyn identified many behaviors that were counterproductive to re-establishing mental health.

One of the most important things we learned from those sessions was that withholding bad news from others, so as not to burden them, wasn't the best strategy to take with family and friends. People can't protect others all the time. My cancer treatment was news that had to be shared, at whatever time and with whatever detail we chose to divulge; let the recipient of the information decide how to handle it. Even exposing our struggles, difficult thoughts and feelings with our children was okay.

Instead of trying to suppress or dismiss sad thoughts, Jocelyn said it was okay to ruminate on them, as long as we only did it for a defined period; when the internal timer sounded, we should learn to put grimness aside until another day. Jocelyn also urged Kathy and me to set aside 15 to 30 minutes every day when each of us in turn could tell the other what was at the top of our minds. And Jocelyn taught us strategies and tactics to prevent simple arguments from escalating into something more unpleasant.

With weekly and bi-weekly visits, it took Kathy and me more than a year to regain some equilibrium.

Normal for me now included having a heavily scarred and occasionally sore abdomen, incontinence requiring the use of underwear pad liners during the day and Depends at night, sexual dysfunction (hello to the blue pill), frequently having cold hands and, worst of all, worrying about recurrence.

National Cancer Survivors Day is an observance scheduled for the first Sunday in June in the U.S. On June 5, 2006, Kathy and I participated in a parade on the athletic fields behind an elementary school near our house. The identifying logo was imprinted on purple T-shirts given to survivors to wear during the walk. But when faced with the prospect of joining a crowd of purple shirt wearers, I couldn't do it. I felt that wearing that shirt meant that cancer defined me. So, I walked awkwardly with the shirt slung over my shoulder. Although that was the only time I participated in a Cancer Survivors Day event, I've continued to support various cancer research activities over the years.

Over time, the worry about recurrence would fade. And it almost disappeared just over a decade later, as I confronted a more dire situation that tested our family's courage and resilience.

# 7

# Before and After

BEING DIAGNOSED WITH a life-threatening cancer bifurcates one's life into a *before* and *after*. With my battle with cancer—and life in the before—now in the rear-view mirror, my family and I began operating in the after. Although I gradually regained confidence, I couldn't completely shed apprehension about my cancer recurring. Because Kathy and my children were keeping a close eye on me, I tried to appear free of worry.

My return to clinical practice was rewarding and invigorating. My new appreciation of what it's like to be a patient led to me to be a better doctor, I think—more focused, more empathetic and more willing to sit and listen whenever verbose patients presented convoluted histories.

Happily, my children seemed none the worse for wear. Patrick progressed nicely through his high school years at Thayer Academy, while Kaylin transitioned from junior high to high school; both continued to do well in their academic and athletic activities. Brendan moved up in elementary school. After five semesters, Dan decided he'd had enough college and found his footing working for a successful residential construction company.

Kathy, the hub of the family spokes, kept everything running as smoothly as possible.

And we expanded our household. Marley, our Bichon Frise, had died, and in 2011, Patrick persuaded Kathy to join him in looking at some puppies being offered at a farm outside Boston. A few days later, I met Mazzy, our new chocolate Labrador puppy. The runt of the litter, she was shy, but adorable. Over many days, Patrick trained her, at times sleeping on our family room floor to calm her while she was whining. Not surprisingly, Mazzy was most attached to Patrick.

A few years later, the stars aligned to add two new members to our extended family. Through a group date with friends in the summer of 2013, Kaylin, who was then teaching kindergarten, met Paul Nimblett, a teacher and coach at Norwood (Massachusetts) High School. They hit it off and the attraction grew. Fearing that her older brothers wouldn't be thrilled about her dating a man eight years her senior, Kay kept their romance a secret for many months. Then one Friday afternoon as I was driving home, Kay called. "Dad," she said, "I think I've found the person for me."

Kathy and I met Paul during a breakfast outing a few weeks later, and we were delighted. The romance flourished for several years. During that time, I learned that Paul had faced a medical crisis in his own family in the summer of 2004 when his father, aged 47—a non-smoker—was diagnosed with nasopharyngeal cancer and underwent aggressive chemotherapy. Although his initial prognosis was positive, he had undetected metastatic disease and died shortly after being diagnosed.

A few months after meeting Paul, we were all on vacation in Cape Cod when he pulled me aside and asked my blessing to marry my daughter. Blessing granted.

Paul decided to propose to Kay during our annual stay at the Atlantis Paradise Island resort, in The Bahamas in August 2016. He wanted to do it after dinner at an outdoor restaurant at the edge of Nassau Harbor. Everyone in our family knew what was coming. When dinner was over,

Amanda suggested that we all gather for a family picture along the water. It was a clear night and the stars shone like diamonds. A gentle, warm breeze wafted among us. Paul got down on one knee and asked Kay to be his wife. Stunned, she started crying—and said yes. Our waiter, who had glasses ready, served us champagne as everyone in the restaurant applauded.

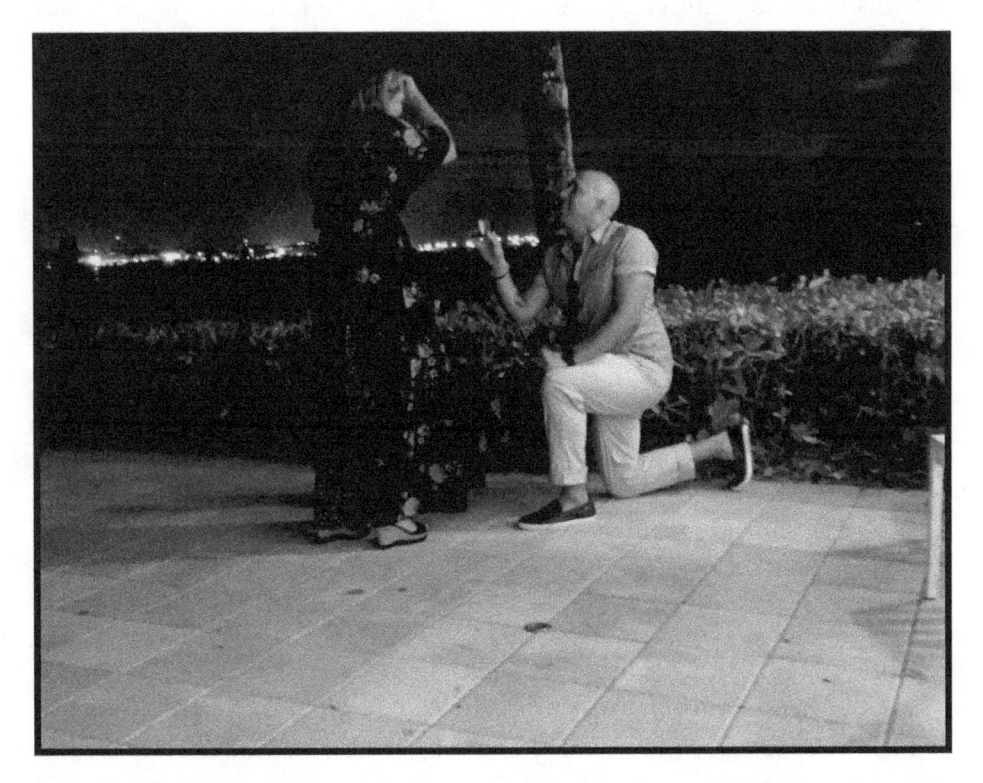

Photo Credit: Melissa Hart

They made plans to marry in just over a year.

Meanwhile, Dan was dating Melissa Burtis Hart, who had grown up in Medfield and known the Beauregard family for years. Melissa graduated from Southern Methodist University's Cox School of Business. She worked in Boston in advertising for a few years and then entered the fashion business in New York City's West Village.

Dan was typically evasive when questioned about girlfriends. One day, a picture surfaced showing Pat, Amanda, Dan and Melissa enjoying an outdoor country western music concert. When asked, Dan acknowledged only that, "She's a friend." Then more pictures of them together began to appear. Finally, Dan informed Kathy and me that they were dating. A few months later, he announced his intent to propose to her. It happened as they stood on a balcony sipping wine at a resort in Sedona, Arizona. Melissa joyfully accepted. Their marriage was planned for the summer of 2019.

During those years, we also lost a member of the extended family. My adoptive father, Rodolphe, who had a long history of smoking, had been diagnosed with kidney cancer in his mid-fifties. Fortunately, his cancer was localized in the right kidney, and he was cured by its removal. He lived to 82, but in his last years, he suffered from dementia and ultimately had to be placed in a long-term nursing facility. When he died in April 2015, Patrick happened to be the sole family member at his bedside. Rudy loved all his grandchildren equally. They called him *Pepere*—an affectionate French term for a grandfather—but Patrick had a special place in his heart because of their shared military service.

It was the first time that Pat saw someone die. He knew the man lying in the bed in front of him was no longer the grandfather he had loved, but fond memories leavened his sadness.

Later, while battling his cancer, Patrick wrote, "I've been thinking a lot about Pepere lately. I was the only one there when he took his last breath. No one should have to suffer and die like that. Alone in a nursing home and not even aware of who you are or who your family is. No proper goodbye. Tomorrow is never promised. I could die tomorrow driving around or crossing the street. People (including myself) take life for granted."

In the personal journal he kept while fighting cancer, Patrick confided that he believed that Pepere was in heaven, and that he would be there waiting for Patrick.

At around the time I reached my early fifties, I started receiving inquiries from national executive search firms asking about my interest in physician-executive roles. The inquiries reflected a transformation going on in health-care delivery to a so-called accountable care or value-based model. Under that system, hospitals and other health-care providers work together while being held accountable for serving distinct populations of patients. The idea is to promote quality and efficiency, providing the right treatment at the right time and avoiding duplication of services. Success is measured in part by health improvements for the population being served and by reduced costs. To oversee these operations, the various networks needed physicians with experience managing health care for large numbers of patients. That's where I came in.

By then, I felt mentally and emotionally ready to transition out of a bustling clinical practice. In late 2009, I accepted an offer from a medium-sized hospital system in southeastern Massachusetts to run its large physician organization. I would be acting for populations now rather than individual patients. I embraced the challenges with enthusiasm.

The inquiries about physician-executive jobs continued to come, and I recognized that I needed professional coaching on how to navigate the opportunities. Someone introduced me to Peter Rabinowitz, the owner of a renowned executive-search firm in Boston. Known as The Rabbi (which he wasn't), he was sought as much for his spiritual advice as for his job expertise.

Rabinowitz had earned a reputation as a seen-it-all change agent in the higher levels of the executive-search world. There was talk of his flamboyant personality and extravagant lifestyle. His signature saying was "Burn with a clear blue flame." Before meeting him, I wasn't sure that we could comfortably work together.

What I didn't know was that, after being diagnosed with prostate cancer at 56 in March 2000 and enduring the side effects of hormone treatments and radiation therapy, he had whittled himself down to his core values and had what others described as "a descent to decency."

In our first meeting, in a tavern restaurant on Cape Cod, we shared our experiences with cancer and moved to such interests as books, authors, television shows, and so on. We bonded immediately. While he was funny, quick-witted and gifted at wordplay, his style of humor could be mordant, as well. Kathy and my children grew fond of him as well. After meeting him for the first time, Kathy described him as a "genie that you can't put back in the bottle." He and his significant other, Judith, joined us for many family events.

After a long remission, Peter's prostate cancer returned and spread to his bones. Over the following years, while he was in his sixties, we had several conversations about the mental struggles associated with having cancer at a fairly young age. We ruminated on such questions as who really knows if they ever get it all? And we wondered if anyone who hasn't had cancer knows what it's like to live without certainty because any new symptom raises the specter of recurrence?

Making a close friend later in life is somewhat of a rarity, so I was grateful. And I was especially grateful to have someone with whom I could share confidences and insights about struggling with cancer.

Peter's mentoring was invaluable, and with his help, I moved from the southeastern Massachusetts system after three years to a system in Harrisburg, Pennsylvania, where I rented an apartment but flew home most weekends. In November 2015, I made a far larger move to a bigger and better opportunity at St. Luke's Health Partners, in Boise, Idaho. Because Dan, Kaylin and Brendan were still living at home, Kathy and I kept our permanent residence in Medfield and rented a condominium near my office in Boise. The change in location was dramatic, but enjoyable. Kathy and I did a lot of hiking, traveling to scenic parts of the state and socializing with new friends. Although it took some getting used to at first, we particularly enjoyed the culture and more laid-back lifestyle of that part of the country.

About every six weeks, we flew back home for vacations and major holidays, and several times the kids visited us. Despite initial howls of protest, Brendan started the second semester of his junior year at Bishop Kelly High School in Boise. As it turned out, the move was transformational for him. He did well, including making friends. But we let him spend his senior year back in Medfield (by then, Kaylin, Paul, and one of my nephews were in the house), setting the stage for him to be accepted to Emerson College, a private liberal-arts college in the heart of Boston. Emerson, recognized for its communications and arts programs, was near where Amanda was working and close to the apartment that she and Patrick were renting in South Boston. Thus, they had frequent opportunities to get together.

Because of my lack of knowledge about the medical histories of my biological parents and my cancer diagnosis at 49, I worried about whether I might carry some genetic abnormality that I had passed on to my children. The Human Genome Project now made testing available—I had an opportunity to meet my genetic profile.

In May 2016, I elected to have a "Multi-Cancer Panel" test done, examining whether I carried a gene associated with cancer. The result came back: *"Negative...No Pathogenic sequence variants or deletions/duplications identified."* I didn't learn whether or not the test results indicated anything about my biological parents, but the possibility of my passing on a dangerous cancer gene to one of my children was unlikely. I breathed a sigh of relief.

But I also thought, who really knows? I would never return to the *before*.

Cancer survivors typically undergo quarterly, bi-annual or annual surveillance testing for their particular cancer. Waiting for the results can be times of enormous stress. Some people call it "scanxiety." For bladder cancer, the tests usually include cystoscopy, but that wasn't indicated for me because my native bladder had been removed. For patients like me, the tests included imaging (in the form of MRIs), certain blood and urine tests and urinary cytology. I started with quarterly office visits and bi-annual

MRIs in Boston, and the tests gradually tapered off. I was tested again after moving to Boise. The tests showed no evidence of recurrence.

In February 2016, after an insurance company rejected my request for supplemental life insurance, my Idaho urologic oncologist, Dr. Stephen Brassell, wrote in a letter to the company: "George Beauregard…is to be considered cured of bladder cancer." To say the least, that statement reassured me. (That notwithstanding, the insurance company still denied me coverage).

Not long after, as if queued up by Dr. Brassell's proclamation, blood reappeared in my urine. While some urine tests showed no evidence of suspicious cells, others showed cells that were "highly suspicious for neoplasm" and "direct visualization" was recommended. Isolated recurrence of urothelial carcinoma within a neobladder without involvement of the upper urinary tract is rare, so no guidelines exist for its management. That prompted a return trip to the operating room. I calmly told Kathy and my children about the situation. On August 30, 2016, I underwent surgery on a tumor in my neobladder and anxiously awaited the biopsy results. Finally, on the day of discharge, Dr. Brassell came by and happily informed me that the tumor was benign—the pathology reports showed no evidence that my cancer was back. As it turned out, that would serve as the last surveillance monitoring I would undergo. The cause of the bleeding remained unknown.

# 8

# "I Will Never Give Up"

AT ONE IN the afternoon on September 14, 2017, I was in my Boise office when I saw that Patrick had left me a text message: "Could you give me a buzz when you have a free minute, please?" A light sense of apprehension came over me. Patrick, then 29, rarely texted me while he knew I was at work. Something was up.

I called him. With a voice sounding slightly tighter than usual and a cadence that just wasn't right, Patrick told me that he had been having intermittent abdominal pain since the previous day—at times severe enough to force him to sit down. The discomfort followed gastrointestinal symptoms—nausea and abdominal pain—that had started after he had lunched with clients the previous day. He later wrote, "I was walking in downtown Boston on my way to my last meeting of the day when a jolt of pain nearly forced me to keel over right on the sidewalk. I walked over to the closest bench I could find, sat down, and took a few breaths to collect myself. I had never experienced pain like this."

His symptoms waxed and waned throughout the rest of the day and led to a poor night's sleep. The next day, he vomited whenever he tried to drink anything. The vomiting somewhat eased the pressure. He decided to stay home that day and call me for advice if things didn't get better by the afternoon.

As he described his situation, I worried most about the tone of his voice. Patrick always had a high pain threshold. What he was describing signaled distress that would've sent most other people to a doctor's office or an emergency room hours earlier. I asked him several routine and "alarm symptom" questions: Did this come on gradually or suddenly? Do you have a fever? Are you having difficulty swallowing? Have you vomited blood? Is your stool bloody or black? On a scale of 1-to-10, with 10 being the worst, what's the level of your pain? Is it constant or intermittent? I also asked if he had experienced any changes in gastrointestinal habits during the preceding months. He said no. He had no reason to suspect that there was something seriously wrong.

Given his answers and the fact that his symptoms had abated somewhat, I told him to take some Tylenol and an antacid, and we'd speak again in an hour or so.

Viral gastroenteritis—particularly Norovirus—topped my list of suspected conditions. Also, given that he had visited Bora Bora and Tahiti a few weeks earlier on his honeymoon, I wondered if he might have contracted some exotic parasitic infection, though I couldn't immediately recall any particular infectious diseases endemic in that part of the world. All in all, our exchange didn't evoke grave concern, and so a diagnostic imperative associated with the signs and symptoms that my son described never crossed my mind.

Because I was scheduled to be in executive meetings for the next couple of hours, I called Kathy and told her about Patrick, and I asked her to call him to see how he was doing and keep me posted.

When she reached him, he sounded very measured but tense, like someone trying to concentrate while riding waves of pain. After hearing his tone and cadence, she told him that he should go to an emergency room as soon as possible and asked him if he felt well enough to take an Uber from the apartment in South Boston to Tufts Medical Center, in downtown Boston. Minutes later, he was en route. Kathy then called Amanda, at work in her law office on Beacon Street not far from the hospital. Amanda said that Patrick had experienced abdominal pain throughout the night before, but he seemed to have improved in the morning. She hadn't heard from him since she left for work, so assumed that he was feeling better. She said she would immediately head to the hospital and asked Kathy to stay home for the time being and wait for updates.

The hospital found no abnormalities on a plain X-ray and laboratory studies, so Patrick was about to be released with a discharge diagnosis of "abdominal pain secondary to constipation" and advice to take Maalox. Suddenly, his vomiting and pain returned, breaking through the medications he had received in the emergency room earlier. The decision to discharge him was canceled. A computerized tomography (CT) scan of his abdomen was ordered. Shockingly, the scan revealed that the cause of Patrick's condition was an obstruction—apparently from a mass lesion evident within his sigmoid colon, the portion of the large intestine just before it reaches the rectum.

Since Patrick had no history of inflammatory bowel disease, the finding was puzzling and alarming. He was kept in the hospital overnight and scheduled to undergo a diagnostic flexible sigmoidoscopy, which would show the lining of the sigmoid colon via a flexible fiber-optic scope. "Cancer was still not mentioned just yet," he later wrote.

The next morning, Kathy went to the hospital and later explained to me what she found and what had happened. Patrick's appearance distressed her. He looked like someone under the influence of narcotic analgesics and trying stoically not to show that he was in significant pain. She accompanied him to the endoscopy suite on the basement floor of the medical center.

With her great intuition, she felt an escalating anxiety. She texted her Aunt Mary Walsh, "For some reason, I have an overwhelming sense of dread. Please God, it can't be cancer. So hopeful that it's not." Her aunt responded, "With you all the way, Kathy. Hopeful, hopeful, hopeful for our strong Patrick. Gran's watching him. Love and hope to Amanda."

The awful feeling eased temporarily when Amanda appeared. She and Kathy embraced in a way that felt very different from the joyous mother and daughter-in-law embraces that they had previously shared. They waited together while Patrick underwent the sigmoidoscopy.

About an hour later, the endoscopy nurse came for them. "The procedure is finished," she said. "Let's go to a room where the doctor can speak to you in private." Fear gripped Kathy. From her years as a hospital-based physical therapist and as the wife of a doctor, she knew that most conversations in doctors' consulting rooms weren't about good news. During those minutes, for the first time, she hated her intuition. Steeling herself, she showed a calm demeanor so as not to alarm Amanda.

They took their place in a small windowless room with a desk and a few chairs. The gastroenterologist, Dr. Mark S, entered a few minutes later. His words were searing. "I never want to pass this information on to anyone, but I have to. I've stented the area of obstruction. I'm certain that the lesion I saw is cancerous." As Amanda started to cry, Kathy hugged her daughter-in-law. A few seconds of silence ensued. It seemed as if the air in the room was getting heavier with each passing second.

"How can you be so sure it's cancer?" Kathy asked finally.

"I imagine you and I are of similar age," the doctor said in a compassionate manner. "I've been doing this for a long time, and I know that what I saw is cancerous. It will be confirmed by the biopsies I took."

Kathy asked Dr. S to tell Patrick of the situation once he had fully recovered from the sedation used in the procedure.

Patrick later wrote, "I remember…hearing the word cancer for the first time." He added that his conversation with the doctor didn't rattle him too much because the initial prognosis was quite positive given how localized the cancer appeared to be. Patrick quickly Googled "colon cancer" to get more information. He saw that the earliest stage colorectal cancers are called stage 0 (a very early cancer that is confined to the innermost lining of the colon and has not spread to deeper layers or nearby lymph nodes). Later stages range from stages I through 4. The lower the number, the less the cancer has spread.

"It brought me hope because at this point we were under the impression I would be officially diagnosed with Stage I or 2," he wrote. He also saw that the current five-year survival rates for lower-stage disease were in the plus 90-percent range. But as he continued reading, he saw that five-year survival rates associated with advanced disease (stage 4) were less than 14 percent.

Kathy kept me apprised of what was happening. I had expected a benign report from the sigmoidoscopy. Using Occam's Razor analysis, I suspected that the findings would show that Patrick had some type of colitis, an inflammation of the colon. A horse, not a zebra. But a zebra diagnosis—say an exotic infection acquired in Tahiti—was possible.

After Kathy spoke to Dr. S, she called me. She sounded tense. "They did Patrick's endoscopy," she said. "The GI doctor is here. I told him he needed to speak to you directly."

A male voice came on the phone. "Dr. Beauregard, this is Dr. S. I've just done a sigmoidoscopy on your son. He's got an apple core lesion in his sigmoid colon. I've taken multiple biopsies, but I'm certain that it's cancer. It's what's causing the obstruction. I've stented it to temporarily relieve that. He'll need to see a surgeon as soon as possible."

His words exploded in my mind. An apple core lesion is the term classically used to describe a malignant, narrowing lesion in the colon.

My mind reeled and my knees buckled as my eyes welled up. *No. No. No. No. NO. NO. NO! How could this be? This can't be. THIS CAN'T BE!* Then: *I've got to pull myself together. For Patrick. For my family. For myself.*

"I'm sure you can understand that I'm shocked at the moment, so I'm struggling for words," I told the doctor. "I'm going to make arrangements to fly back to Boston as soon as possible. Thank you very much for caring for my son. May I speak with my wife again, please?"

I told Kathy that I would get on the next available flight home and said: "Don't worry. Everything will turn out okay." I truly believed what I said then. But at the same time, I understood that putting the advice that I'd offered to hundreds of patients of not catastrophizing medical adversity into practice wasn't going to be easy.

Having a child diagnosed with cancer is a parent's nightmare. In an instant, you become a different person, uncertain whether you'll ever feel joy again. Even worse is the feeling that there's nothing you can do to alter the situation, aside from supporting the child as much as you can. A parent's protective urge is embedded deep in our character, it's instinctive. When cancer strikes your child, you are helpless. It upends the natural order of life.

Kathy called Patrick's siblings, alerting them to their brother's condition and asking them to get to Tufts Medical Center as soon as possible. They arrived together quickly. Brendan, then 18, said that during the ride, he had flashbacks about when I was struck by cancer in 2005. He knew he had to keep it together for his brother. Kaylin later recalled thinking that what people were telling her didn't seem real—they were describing things that weren't really happening. Dan remembered, "I never believed the diagnosis originally. Or maybe I just refused to hear it. My brother had cancer.... Unfathomable."

The next morning, I left the Boise Airport at 5:30. As wonderful as Boise is, it can be hard to get to and from by air. There are no direct flights to the East Coast. The first leg of the 2,600-mile trip typically stops in Chicago, Minneapolis or Phoenix. During the nearly two years that I had been working in Boise, I had regularly flown back to Boston. What I had never done, however, was spend nearly the whole trip staring out of the window in a numbed silence and trying not to cry. I spent the majority of that time trying to figure out how I could be just his father now. For me, medicine was as intrinsic as fatherhood.

Delta Flight 622 arrived in Boston on time. I took an Uber to Tufts Medical Center, arriving there at about 3:30 p.m. and hurried to Patrick's room. I found Amanda's parents, Charlie and Rosalyn (Roz), along with one of Amanda's younger sisters, Devin, outside the door. We briefly embraced before I entered. Patrick was lying in bed, his slippered feet slightly protruding from the sheets and blankets. Amanda was standing nearby, and Kathy sat to his left. I focused on my son's intense hazel eyes as I walked over and hugged him. I asked how he was doing.

He said that he was doing okay. A CT scan of his chest, a standard test recommended for patients with colorectal cancer to help determine the extent of disease, had been done earlier that day. The results hadn't yet come back.

Patrick and Amanda did their best to remain optimistic. "Well, this will certainly make for quite a story to tell our kids someday," Pat jokingly said. "The time Dad had a cancer scare one month after Mom and Dad got married. Talk about 'in sickness and in health.'"

Moments later came a knock on the door.

A man wearing an attending physician's neatly pressed long white coat, entered the room. The words "Dr. James Y, Department of Surgery" were sewn in black cursive on his coat. Dr. Y first introduced himself to Patrick. After other introductions, he said, "I'd like to examine and speak with Patrick, so I'll ask that everyone else leave the room for a few moments. I'll call you back when I'm done." He was professional and polite. To me, he didn't seem to evoke grave concern.

We joined Amanda's parents and Devin in the hallway and talked in hushed tones. Before that day, Kathy and I had enjoyed a friendly though casual relationship with Charlie and Roz Flood. We saw them on certain family occasions. Charlie worked as a senior account executive for an office furniture company and had a calm demeanor and a great sense of humor.

He'd grown up in a family of six children in Lowell, Massachusetts, where the Flood family currently lived. Roz grew up in Michigan, then Florida. She was a paraprofessional for the Lowell public schools and was always good-natured with Kathy and me. Amanda was the oldest of their three daughters. Kathy and I knew the Floods loved Patrick and what he brought to the family as a man. I sensed that our relationship with them was about to get deeper.

While we waited in the hall, Kathy told me that Jack E had come by to see Patrick, and she said that his comments to our son were somewhat encouraging. "I've looked at the abdominal CT scan from yesterday. Your liver looks fine. Hopefully the tumor is well contained. It'll be removed. You will need some standard chemotherapy following that. This could end up being a blip on the screen for you."

After many minutes went by, Dr. Y asked Amanda, Kathy and me to come back into Patrick's room. The first thing we saw were tears streaming down Patrick's face.

"I'd like everyone to sit down," Dr. Y said.

"I always prefer to stand," Kathy told him.

"You really need to sit."

Kathy sat.

Amanda immediately went to the bedside to be near her distraught husband. A mere month before, they had been the centerpiece of a joyful wedding ceremony on Cape Cod, with their future seeming limitless. That already felt as if it had happened a long time ago.

"I'm afraid that I've got some unexpected news about Patrick," Dr. Y explained. The chest CT scan showed that there are multiple nodules—abnormal growths—in both of his lungs. "From the appearance of those nodules, it most likely means the cancer has spread beyond the colon and to his lungs. We won't know for sure until we have some biopsy results, but he likely has stage 4 disease."

Crushing silence followed. Life as we knew it before was over.

Dr. Y told Patrick that he would need to see an oncologist. And he'd need surgery. "While the stent has relieved your symptoms, it can't stay in long, so you'll need to have the tumor removed as quickly as possible. From the CT, the tumor does appear to be confined to the sigmoid region. I think I'll be able to immediately reconnect the areas that the cancer is between, so you probably won't need a colostomy bag. I'm able to do it here if you choose. We can get you on the operating room schedule within a few days. You're in good hands. We'll take very good care of you. Of course, you certainly could seek to have that done by someone else at another hospital. Do you have any questions?"

Hearing none, he said "I'll have my resident come by later today to see how you want to proceed." With that, he quietly left the room.

Later, Patrick wrote, "When the doctor came in and asked my family to leave the room for a moment, I knew something was wrong. You obviously can't prepare yourself for news like that. I completely broke down and shut down. Everything became a blur. Oncologists were called in and the grim diagnosis was officially cast: incurable.

"I felt like everyone who saw me the rest of that day looked at me with such sadness and sorrow, like I was marked dead."

For a few seconds after Dr. Y left, I stood very still, trying to process what I had just heard. While I had begun to expect that Patrick might have stage 2, or at worst stage 3, disease, which could probably be cured by surgery and adjuvant chemotherapy, I had never considered the possibility of stage 4, for which no curative therapy existed. Tears trickled down my cheeks. But I knew that this was not the time to lose it in front of my son, wife, and daughter-in-law.

I struggled to find words of comfort for Patrick. Although I knew that hope is not an element within a statistical probability equation, I had seen how hope in its own way could be a kind of miracle drug—raising the quality of life of some very sick patients and even improving the chances of surviving longer. I put my hands on the sides of Patrick's face and looked into his eyes. "Pat, I know this is not the news you wanted to hear," I told him. "Keep this in mind: You are young. You are strong, physically and psychologically. You are otherwise healthy. You have to stay positive. We have to stay positive. This family has done this before. You were an important part of that. Your positivity and continued efforts to do the best at what you were doing at the time in high school, helped me focus on beating my cancer and becoming a survivor. We can—and will—do it again. I will not lose a son. You will beat this. You will be a survivor. I wish I didn't have to share this wish with you, but we'll be survivors together."

Later that day, the on-call oncologist came by the hospital room and spoke with us. Essentially, he told Patrick that it would be "irresponsible" for him, or anyone else, to say that they could cure him. Making what was already a bad encounter worse, his expression suggested that the situation was hopeless. One of the greatest challenges facing doctors is finding a balance between realism and hope in conversations with very ill patients. Some physicians are adept at it, others not. As unintentional as this oncologist's remarks may have been, they were thoroughly insensitive. As far as we were concerned, he couldn't leave the room fast enough.

Remarkably, though, that encounter ignited Patrick's determination to conquer the cancer. "When the doctor said that it would be irresponsible to say that they could cure this cancer, I felt destroyed," he wrote. "I also knew then that I did not want him treating me. I cannot judge him, but how can you put your life in the hands of someone with no hope? Not me. I refuse. I refuse to lay down like some dog and just die. I will fight with every ounce of my mind and body.

"*I will never give up.*"

Two years later, the memory of that encounter continued to drive Patrick. "I remember everything about that doctor: his face, the way he talked to me and looked at me—hopeless. He was the coldest and most grim man I've ever met. I still use him, and this moment, as motivation when I feel tired of fighting."

As I reflected on the news of that day, I recalled that during my more than 20 years as a practicing physician, I had seen many surprising outcomes. In some, patients with serious medical conditions with high statistical chances of recovery had died prematurely from their illness. In others, patients with poor prognoses survived well beyond what had been anticipated based on the medical evidence.

I remembered two patients in particular: one diagnosed with a rare form of a neuro endocrine cancer whose hospice care was discontinued several times over a couple years because she was independently functional and doing fine. Another patient was an elderly man who was brought to the emergency department in a totally unresponsive state because of a non-hemorrhagic stroke. Tests showed minimal brain activity. Days passed with his condition unchanged. The thought of him coming back to life was like expecting a rock to start walking and talking. But suddenly he awoke and eventually left the hospital with no residual cognitive or physical deficits.

Once again, I found myself thinking of survival rates as a two-sided coin and hoped that my son would come up heads—among the 1% of those with his stage 4 cancer who survive for 10 years.

Grim as that statistic was, I knew it was calculated from patient populations that were older (aged 55–75). How the rates pertained to my 29-year-old son was uncertain. I knew the mortality statistics in older people would be higher because some of them die from competing causes—such as heart disease and diabetes—not directly related to CRC. I also knew younger people were more likely to die from the disease itself. At the same time, rapid advances in therapies were emerging, so survival rates could easily improve.

September 18, 2017, was the one-month anniversary of Patrick and Amanda's wedding. Rather than a day of celebration, it was the day Patrick underwent surgery by Dr. Y at Tufts Medical Center. The immediate members of the Beauregard and Flood families gathered in a small waiting area outside the operating-room suites. The conversation was desultory. A television droned news. About an hour after the start of the surgery, comfort food arrived from Maggiano's Little Italy, one of Boston's famous Italian restaurants, courtesy of some of Amanda's co-workers at the law firm.

After another hour or so, Dr. Y appeared. He asked Kathy, Amanda, and me to follow him to a small waiting room. A single framed picture hung on one of the walls—a photo of three Pandas in their natural environment. It seemed to radiate hope. After all, Patrick and Amanda were collectively nicknamed Panda.

Dr. Y told us that the operation had gone well. He had removed about six inches of Patrick's sigmoid colon and reconnected the remaining segments without complications. Additionally, 25 lymph nodes within the area of the cancer were also removed. Some were immediately cut into thin slices and frozen to be examined under a microscope by a pathologist. Those results would inform the surgeon if additional surgery was needed. Fortunately, the specimens did not reveal the presence of cancer. Patrick's post-op course was uneventful, and he was discharged after a few days.

Patrick and Amanda returned to their apartment in South Boston. Within a couple of weeks, he resumed work, albeit in a hybrid manner—partly remote and partly in the office. His near future included more tests as well as finding an oncologist with expertise in colorectal cancer—and a bedside manner that appealed to him and Amanda.

One early test was the Positron Emission Tomography (PET) scan, an imaging test used for diagnosing numerous diseases. A PET scan uses a mildly radioactive drug to highlight areas of the body where higher levels of cellular activity are occurring. Compared to normal cells, cancer cells are hyperactive. Patrick's PET scan was followed by a bronchoscopy—a look inside the lungs via a bronchoscope, a thin, flexible tube with a light and a small video camera on the end. Several biopsies of some of the lung nodules and lymph nodes were taken. The reports of those images and samples came back confirming the presence of cancer. Our worst fears were realized. The diagnosis of stage 4 disease was now confirmed. But I kept telling myself, "He will beat this. I will not lose one of my sons. I won't let that happen."

As he had only seen the covering oncologist during his hospital stay, Patrick needed to see a different oncologist as quickly as possible. I could help in finding the right one. I knew that the current first-line standard of chemotherapy care for stage 4 colorectal cancer (CRC) was well established. The problem was that the treatment options were limited—there wasn't a plethora of effective drugs. As dear as Jack E was to us as a physician and a trusted adviser, his expertise was in breast cancer. So, he recommended a colleague at Tufts with an international reputation. Patrick and Amanda consented to having Kathy and me present during the consultation.

The meeting didn't go well from the start. The doctor walked into the room wearing a foam neck collar, which obscured the lapels of his long white coat. After a cursory introduction, he began speaking at length about the after-effects of a recent car accident he had been in. Patrick and Amanda tried their best to hide their irritation. After the doctor finally gave his opinion about Pat's cancer and how to treat it, he called Patrick "my friend" and told him that he would give Pat his cell phone number, so "you can call me anytime." I didn't think I was alone in sensing his insincerity. Patrick and Amanda felt that although the physician's clinical expertise in treating colorectal cancer may have been impressive, his bedside manner was incompatible with what they were looking for. For Patrick, strike two on the oncology doc front.

As a practicing physician, I had an immediately available mental Rolodex of expert colleagues in many different specialties—an advantage I wish existed for everyone with urgent medical conditions. Through St. Luke's, I knew a Boise-based oncologist named Dan Zuckerman, who specialized in gastrointestinal malignancies, particularly colorectal cancer. He recommended a former colleague—Kimmie Ng, an expert in colorectal cancer currently working at the famed Dana-Farber Cancer Institute in Boston. I was a bit apprehensive at first—Dana-Farber was where I'd seen the oncologist who'd told me the wolf was out of the cage. Still, I had great confidence in Zuckerman. Although Dr. Ng couldn't see every patient referred to her, given that Dan was her friend and I was a colleague of his, she agreed to see Patrick; an appointment was scheduled for within a week.

On October 18, Patrick, Amanda, Kathy and I gathered at the Gastrointestinal Cancer Center at Dana-Farber for the initial consultation with Dr. Ng. As we walked into the large waiting room, I noticed other patients looking at Patrick—he appeared so healthy and alive. Were they thinking that Kathy or I was the patient? They quickly found out when they spotted his Dana-Farber ID bracelet or saw him being summoned by a receptionist behind a glass-partitioned cubicle. The four of us were led to an exam room, and after a few minutes, following a gentle knock on the door, Dr. Ng entered. She first greeted Patrick, who was seated on the exam table, and then the rest of us.

Dr. Ng was slender and graceful and stood about 5 feet, 6 inches tall. She had a calm, focused demeanor and radiated measured compassion. She listened to Patrick's answers to her inquiries without interruption.

She then pulled up images from his CT scan on her computer monitor. The initial image of a CT scan typically shows a collection of individual two-dimensional images known as slices, which show the inside of the patient's body arranged sequentially. She began scrolling down the slices until she arrived at the most important views of both of his lungs. She pointed to and described the number, sizes and shapes of the numerous pulmonary nodules present and reviewed his most recent lab results. Then she walked through his chemotherapy options.

While I felt that she wasn't sugarcoating anything, I also sensed that she was trying to have Patrick, Amanda and the rest of us maintain some hope, unlike the other oncologists who had evaluated Pat.

Listening to an oncologist talk to one of my children was eerie. As a doctor, I'd seen hundreds of CT scan images. With limited compassion, I looked at them through the detached lens of a clinical diagnostician. In the past, what I'd seen, one slice at a time, were just grayscale pixels forming tissues and organs, some normal appearing, others looking hideously abnormal. When necessary, I would call on a radiologist to review a scan.

What I saw during that visit with Dr. Ng, in what seemed like slow motion, weren't just two-dimensional, static images of seemingly inanimate objects. They had become multiple aggressive living mutations with an insatiable desire to destroy all cells they encountered in my son's lungs and elsewhere.

When the session was over, I felt some relief that Patrick was in expert and compassionate hands. Importantly, Patrick and Amanda liked Dr. Ng's bedside manners. But that didn't alleviate my deep concern about the ravages of chemotherapy and dismal treatment success rates.

Before his consultation with Dr. Ng, Patrick had undergone a number of tests to more precisely profile the nature of his cancer. Even within the general diagnosis of colon cancer, the malignancy can have differing biologic and genetic characteristics. Identifying them helps target the best chemotherapy and immunotherapy drugs to use.

During the consultation, Dr. Ng went over Patrick's routine lab results. To begin with, I was surprised that most, if not all of Patrick's tests came back within normal ranges. In particular, a test for a small protein produced by about 90 percent of colorectal cancers—the Carcinogenic Embryonic Antigen (CEA)—came back negative. A false negative. That told me that if Patrick were to achieve remission, it wasn't clear how effective testing for CEAs would be in detecting recurrence.

Samples of Patrick's tumor had undergone Next Generation Sequencing (NGS), a technology used for testing tumor DNA and RNA sequencing and variant mutations. This technology looks for, and interrogates, specific genetic mutations in the cancer's DNA along with the tumor mutation burden associated with it. The test also helps identify different mutation targets for targeted therapy. The tests showed alterations in several genes contained within his tumor.

This news wasn't good. One of the oncogenes—cancer-causing genes—in Patrick's tumor was the so-called KRAS (for Kirsten ras sarcoma viral oncogene homologue). The KRAS gene, one of the most highly mutated oncogenes in human cancer, occurs in about 30 to 40 percent of colorectal carcinomas. When KRAS is mutated, it becomes permanently activated. Patients whose tumors express the mutation do not respond to specific targeted therapies, such as certain immunotherapy drugs known to be effective against colorectal cancer cells.

In addition, Patrick's tumor had what's known as microsatellite stability (MSS). A microsatellite represents a short sequence of DNA repeated together in a row along the DNA molecule. Colorectal cancers with MSS respond poorly to the immunotherapy drugs that have been game changers for other malignancies, such as lung cancer and melanoma.

So where did that leave Patrick? Until the 1990s, the mainstay of chemotherapy for the treatment of stage 2 to stage 4 colorectal cancer was fluorouracil (known as 5-FU). Often it is taken with folinic acid, which enhances 5-FU's effect. Since 2017, various combinations of 5-FU and other anti-cancer drugs have been the backbone of treatment. The other drugs include oxaliplatin (a platinum-based alkylating agent considered the most neurotoxic chemotherapy), and irinotecan. Depending on the combination and how many drugs are included, the drug regimen is known as FOLFOX, FOLFIRI or FOLFOXIRI. Among them, FOLFOXIRI would in theory be the strongest against cancer, but also the harshest to the patient.

While various chemotherapeutic drugs have different mechanisms to attack cancer cells, chief among the means are the disruption of certain DNA-related activities. So 5-FU works by interfering with the synthesis in the cell of DNA and RNA (ribonucleic acid), which helps pass on instructions for growth from DNA.

Oxaliplatin, once it enters the cell, binds to the DNA of the cancer cells and produces what are known as "adducts"—abnormal DNA structures that inhibit downstream replication. As a result, the cell cycle (whereby the cell copies itself) is arrested and the cell eventually dies. Interestingly, oxaliplatin also affects the DNA repair mechanisms within the cancer cells, further contributing to the cell death process.

Irinotecan works by inhibiting a specific molecular enzyme, leading to an unwinding and separating of DNA strands. In the end, both agents disrupt DNA replication, eventually leading to cell death.

Dr. Ng recommended one type of immunotherapy drug that could work against Patrick's cancer. Bevacizumab (brand name Avastin) is designed to block a protein that promotes the growth of new blood vessels that feed tumors. Unlike chemotherapy, which attacks cancer cells, Avastin's purpose is to block the blood supply that feeds the tumor, which can stop the tumor from growing.

In the end, Dr. Ng laid out the choices for Patrick—FOLFOX, FOLFIRI or FOLFOXIRI—and left it for him to decide how to proceed.

Dr. Ng could be helpful in another way, too. As a researcher, she was knowledgeable about the various clinical trials underway and about to start in Boston and across America. These are trials where new and evolving treatments can be tested on consenting patients. My advice to any people affected by atypical cancers is do whatever it takes to see a clinician researcher. Your survival might depend on it.

I was raised as a Roman Catholic. While I tried to live my life following Christian values, I was never devout. With what was now happening with my son, I was angry at God. To me, Patrick's situation was another sign that, at best, God was indifferent to bad things happening to good people.

In contrast, Patrick had maintained his faith, and he and Amanda were regular church goers. As his treatment was about to begin, Patrick evoked a homily attributed to Padre Pio, an Italian friar, saint and mystic: *"Pray, hope and don't worry. Worry is useless. God is merciful and will hear your prayer."* In 2002, 14 years after Padre Pio's death at 81, Pope John Paul II declared him a saint for his piety and charity. Patrick said he would rely on Padre Pio's homily as an inspiration during his treatment journey. Kathy custom-ordered light-gray rubber wristbands. On half of the band were the words *"Panda Power."* The other half read *"Pray, Hope, Don't Worry."* Within weeks, hundreds of people were wearing the bands.

Later, Patrick and Amanda used email and social media to organize friends and family into Team Panda, a support group that helped raise thousands of dollars for cancer research. Soon the wristbands were joined by T-shirts, sweatshirts and hats that bore Padre Pio's inspiring words.

Given the extent of the healthcare services Patrick was about to receive, I wondered whether his health insurance would cover the treatment. The average cost of one year of treatment for advanced colon cancer was about $30,000.

Both Kathy and I had extensive experience in dealing with local and national health insurers. Such things as plan designs, pharmacy benefits, provider networks, co-insurance and deductibles were familiar to us. Typically, people can only change health plans during open enrollment periods. Many health plans, however, have special enrollment criteria that let people retroactively change insurance coverage within 30 days of getting married. On Kathy's suggestion, Patrick disenrolled as a subscriber to his current health plan (which covered certain veterans) and became a dependent on Amanda's plan, which we knew would offer a much broader provider network and expenditures coverage.

Nonetheless, the insurance situation was overwhelming for Patrick and even confounded Amanda, who was a health-care lawyer. They didn't have a good sense from the beginning of what they owed to whom and they felt as if they were playing catch up for a long time. On top of that, Amanda's plan had a $6,000 deductible—meaning that the policyholder is responsible for the first $6,000 of expenses before the insurance carrier pays anything. Fortunately, generous donors covered nearly all of their deductible amount.

Another pre-treatment issue: Chemotherapy can destroy reproductive cells. Because Patrick and Amanda wanted to have children, Kathy advised Patrick to bank some of his sperm before chemotherapy, which he did. For her part, Amanda underwent the initial steps of In-vitro fertilization.

Eggs were taken from her ovaries for the purpose of combining them with sperm. If successful, that process results in a fertilized egg (an embryo), which would eventually be placed in her uterus and result, if things went well, in a pregnancy. Undaunted, Patrick and Amanda chose to create three embryos, the number of children they wanted.

Following his initial visit with Dr. Ng, Patrick had to decide which of the treatment regimens he'd receive. Otherwise healthy and active patients like him are believed to be able to tolerate aggressive combination chemotherapy—so-called doublet chemotherapy, with 5-FU and another drug, or triplet chemotherapy with 5-FU, oxaliplatin, and irinotecan. Patrick and I discussed the available research and the impact of treatment on his quality of life. At the time, some modest evidence suggested that first-line FOLFOXIRI—the full blast triplet—provided a clinically meaningful benefit, but at the expense of increased toxicity. Patrick chose that regimen, along with the immunotherapy drug Avastin. I agreed with his choice.

About the decision, Patrick later wrote in CaringBridge, "Having a confirmed Stage 4 diagnosis, we began to explore treatment options. The standard chemotherapy drugs for colon cancer were well established, having been around for a while.... [We chose] the most powerful and effective as possible. More toxic. More side effects. Lower quality of life.... I was 29 years old and felt like my life was just starting, there was no way I wasn't going to fight as hard as possible."

The duration of chemotherapy treatment, given in cycles, for people with stage 4 colorectal cancer varies from months to years. So, the plan was for Patrick to go as long as he could, based on his ability to tolerate side effects, while the effectiveness of the treatment was assessed via serial scans. Blood tests—looking for adverse effects on his blood cell counts, liver and kidneys—would be part of that plan as well. It was a daunting prospect.

People undergoing certain types of chemotherapy get what's known as a port-a-cath to provide long-term access to the bloodstream and avoid repeated punctures of peripheral veins. A small disc (the port) is inserted under the skin—typically in the chest. A catheter (a thin flexible tube) is connected. One end of the catheter is advanced into a large vein while the other end is connected to the port—hence the port-a-cath. Shortly after the initial visit with Dr. Ng and before starting chemotherapy, Patrick underwent the implantation of a port-a-cath under local anesthesia.

Kaylin and Paul had long ago set their wedding for November 2017. Patrick started treatment about three weeks before, at the end of October. "The first time I got chemo is something I'll never forget," he later wrote. "Sitting in that chair (which smells like strong cleaning products and still makes me sick to this day) and seeing the bag of toxic chemicals slowly drip into your body. You sit there and tell yourself it is medicine, and it is helping you. But it sucks. Bad. You sit there for hours looking at your wife, your parents, your family. Thinking. Hoping. Praying. I tried to imagine myself in their shoes and I was glad to be the one sitting in the chair.

"Dana-Farber has a good system where they try to pair you with one infusion nurse that you see every time you come in for infusion appointments. They seem to try to match you based on age, interests, etc. We ended up getting paired up with Taylor, and it was great. Taylor was a blessing for us because she really tried her hardest to make those sessions as easy, comfortable and as exciting as she could. She was often a welcome distraction with her funny stories and comments. Those infusion nurses are the real heroes—caring for these patients' day in and day out; and always doing it with a smile on their faces. It is (obviously) not the most fun work environment to be in, so I give them all the credit in the world."

Patrick bounced back quickly from his first round of chemo. He continued with his job and worked out at the gym. He and Amanda spent a fun weekend in Providence, in part walking around the Providence College campus, reliving old memories. Despite the trauma of his diagnosis, he confided in his journal, "There are times when I forget that I have cancer."

He had his second round of chemotherapy two weeks after the first, and just a few days before Kaylin's wedding. That round hit harder. "I'm just not feeling myself today," he wrote. "I wish I could just snap out of it but it's not that easy. I feel tired and worn down. It's hard to describe the way that chemo makes you feel. I just don't really feel like myself."

He wrote those comments in his private journal on Veterans Day, adding that it's "important to think of all the sacrifices our veterans, past and present, have made for us." But then he continued in a gloomier vein, regretting that he hadn't had a more active role during his Marine service. "I wish I could've served my country the way I intended to. It looks unlikely now that I would be able to return and serve, but I pray I get the opportunity again. Becoming a Marine is one of the proudest moments of my life. No one can take that title from you and you've earned it."

# 9

# Chemo Days

THE WEDDING OF our only daughter, Kaylin Marguerite Beauregard, to Paul Westlin Nimblett Jr. took place on November 18 in a lovely, restored old mill along the Chocheco River in Dover, New Hampshire. For the first time since Patrick's diagnosis had hung its heavy cloak on our entire family, we had a day filled with happiness.

Kaylin and I have quite different personalities. I'm calm, rather stoic and have OCD—performing certain routines repetitively, such as leveling crooked wall hangings or puffing sofa cushions. She's a bit anxious, impulsive and messy. As she and I waited for the walk down the aisle, she looked beautiful in her wedding dress. But she whispered to me, "I don't know if I can walk down the aisle with everyone staring at me."

I gripped her hand. "You most certainly can do this," I told her. "They're all here for you. This is your day."

She managed the walk with consummate elegance. Awaiting us at the front were Paul, looking a bit nervous though joyful himself, and the officiant, my best friend, Bob Neidermire, the father of Kay's best friend,

Kim, who was maid of honor. I took a seat at Kathy's side in the front row. Kathy beamed with joy, as did our entire family and virtually everyone else there for the occasion.

After the ceremony, a festive evening followed, filled with good food and drinks, a lot of laughter and dancing. Kaylin grabbed my heart with the father-daughter dance song she'd picked, "Make You Feel My Love," by Adele, a favorite of both of ours. To this day, whenever the song comes up on my playlist, I fight back the tears.

My friend Peter Rabinowitz and his significant other, Judith, attended the ceremony. At the time, Peter was undergoing chemotherapy treatments for his relapsed metastatic prostate cancer. Compared to when I last saw him several months before, he looked terrible. The twinkle in his eye was still there, but dimmer. He had to use a cane when walking.

I frequently glanced toward Patrick, who had recently completed his second round of chemotherapy. He and Amanda seemed full of living-in-the-moment joy and laughter. I saw the same spontaneous pleasure in the rest of the family. Once again, outshone by the light of a joyful event, cancer's darkness had relaxed its vise-like grip on our family. But only temporarily.

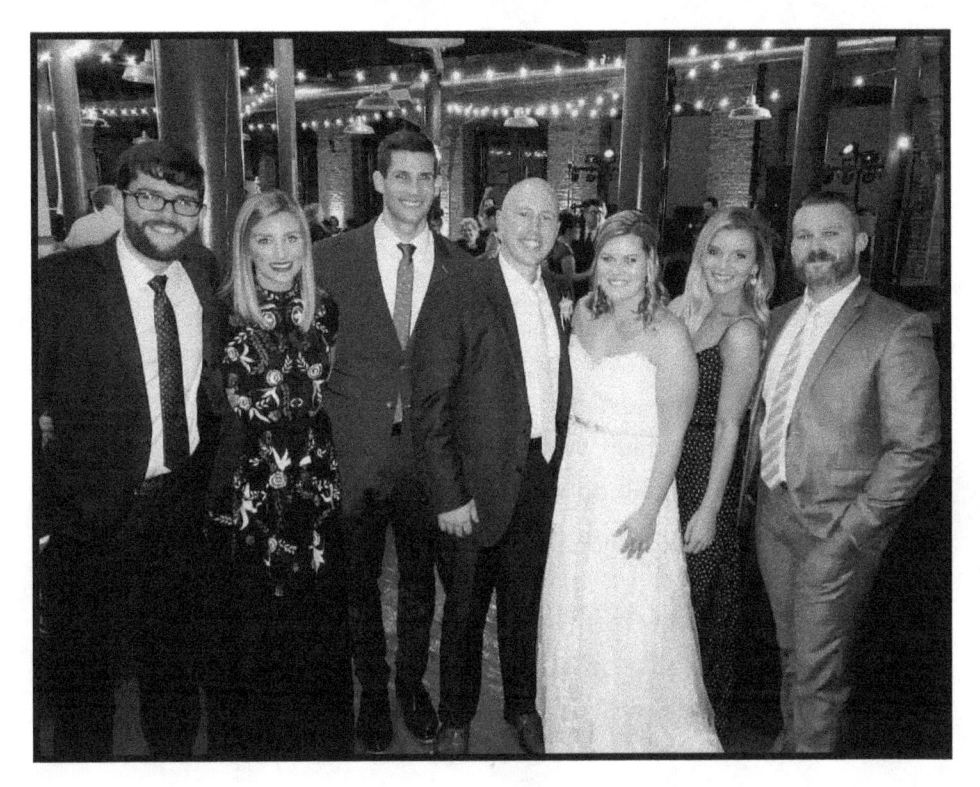

Photo Credit: Eric McCallister

Later, Patrick wrote, "We all had a great weekend at Kay and Paul's wedding. Paul is truly a great, caring and genuine guy. Kaylin seemed very happy, and that's all that matters." He said it recalled his own wedding with Amanda. "I wish I could go back and relive that all over again. It was such a fun, happy weekend."

Patrick saw that Peter Rabinowitz seemed to be struggling, both mentally and physically. "His chemo treatment seems to be taking a serious toll on him. I need to send him a card to let him know I'll be praying and thinking of him. It makes me feel horrible to see someone struggling and suffering like that.

"All I know is that I can't let this get to me mentally like that. Regardless of what news I receive next month after my scan, I can't get disheartened, and I can't ever give up.

"Never give up."

"I think my dad said it best the other day: Once you get diagnosed with cancer it's like putting on a coat or cloak that can never come off. Even if I beat this and show no signs of disease, this will always stay with me and always be in the back of my mind. My life was forever changed last September."

Patrick's chemotherapy was arduous. He went into Dana-Farber every other Wednesday to get blood work, see Dr. Ng or her nurse practitioner, and then get the chemo infusions. They were long days, six to eight hours.

Kathy and I usually met him and Amanda there. I think that he appreciated the presence of his parents, mostly because he understood what it entailed for us in terms of logistics. He hated people staring at him, which we didn't do. He sometimes listened to music, other times he read. He frequently napped. Amanda and I worked on our laptops. Kathy usually brought magazines. There was a lot of casual conversation. As a reminder of life outside the infusion center, Patrick and Amanda had a small routine of setting up a cadre of items—pictures of family and Padre Pio, and other items for good luck—on a stand by his chair.

Because the infusion time for 5-FU stretched over about 48 hours and needed to proceed slowly, he would leave the clinic connected to a portable infusion pump, which featured a small motor that repeatedly made what Pat described as a haunting, whirring noise. He had to learn how to properly disconnect and dispose of the chemo drug bag, remove the needle from the port in his chest, then inject himself with saline solution to flush out the port before returning the pump to Dana-Farber.

At home, Patrick had to give himself a shot to keep up his blood count. Though chemotherapy fights cancer cells, it also affects other operations of the body. Among them is the production of blood cells by rapidly dividing cells in bone marrow. Accordingly, patients on chemotherapy need to have their blood cell counts monitored frequently to watch for serious reductions. If the cells that fight infections—neutrophils—decline significantly, the patient faces an increased susceptibility to infections and other complications.

Predictably, Patrick's neutrophil count decreased while he was on chemotherapy, so he needed to give himself a shot of a so-called growth factor medication (pegfilgrastim, brand name Neulasta), which increases the number of neutrophils in the body. "If you've never had to inject yourself, it's weird," he wrote. "You become numb to it after a while."

As the cycles progressed, Patrick found that the early rounds weren't all that bad. "The long days were draining, but the side effects were minimal at first," he wrote in CaringBridge, the social media blog he and Amanda posted for family and friends. "Rounds 1–10 felt somewhat like a breeze. We were expecting much worse. Not like there weren't any side effects. Typically, the Friday after going into Dana-Farber (the day I disconnected from the 5-FU bag) and the following Saturday were pretty miserable. I wouldn't do much moving from the couch, and eating and drinking became increasingly difficult.

"They warned us up front—the more chemo you do, the worse it gets. The side effects are cumulative. There is only so much detoxing the body can do. We quickly began to notice that I wasn't bouncing back nearly as fast as I was in the earlier rounds. The feeling of being miserable was starting to extend into Sunday. And then into Monday."

As more treatment cycles went by, Patrick's state of mind slumped occasionally along with his physical decline. On December 28, 2017, he wrote in his private journal, "The fear of being forgotten weighs much more heavily on me than the actual thought of death itself. I keep thinking that I will die, and then a couple of years later I am just some afterthought to my family and friends. It's a sad reality but it's the truth. People get caught up in their own lives and move on. I'd just become a fleeting memory to people every so often and that scares me.

"I don't ever want to take my time on this earth for granted ever again. Thank God every morning and every night for another day and all the blessings He has given me." Patrick cited a quote he'd read from someone dying from breast cancer: "It no longer matters to me how long I live. What matters to me most is how I live."

The platinum-based chemo drugs are considered to be highly effective against various types of cancer but can leave you feeling like a wreck and damage parts of the body not directly affected by the cancer, including the kidneys, the nervous system, bone marrow, and the gastrointestinal system. Patrick took oxaliplatin, a drug he called "an absolute beast."

The news that my son was going to receive this drug resurfaced my haunting memory of cisplatin, the platinum-based drug I took for my bladder cancer. During the four months that I was taking it, I'd never felt so awful in my life. I'll never forget the loss of taste, profound fatigue, nausea and the "chemo brain" effects I experienced. Although Patrick wasn't one to linger on how chemotherapy was affecting him, he and I occasionally talked about our shared experience with the treatment. Mostly, I tried to reassure him that those side effects were to be expected—and would disappear once he was done with treatment.

Patrick described the torment he was going through in an entry in CaringBridge. "As the rounds mounted, we were granted a few breaks here and there. Even a week extension break from chemo was truly a blessing. I can't describe how hard it was to wake up on those chemo Wednesdays. I hated going into that place. I started getting nauseous just driving in there, so much so that I had to start taking anti-nausea and anti-anxiety medication just to get myself through the door. I hated the way chemo was making me feel, and I hated how useless I felt. I'd be embarrassed to see Amanda working all day and coming home to clean and cook to try to force feed me something (exactly what I needed) when I couldn't even get off the couch.

"Days on the chemo bag became a total blur. I began sleeping probably 75% of the day. I couldn't eat. My appetite was almost completely gone now for extended periods of time after each round. I weighed 195 pounds at the time of my diagnosis. I was 163 pounds after chemo. The lack of appetite was probably my worst side effect. Eating became an act of revulsion. Food would taste like hot/cold mushy cardboard.

"Thankfully, I had Amanda by my side helping me through it the entire time. It is damn impossible to stir up that motivation and fight inside of you all by yourself day in and day out. You need someone/something, whatever it may be for you, to be there. Thankfully, I have Amanda, I have the best family I could ever ask for, and I have the best friends and an army of incredible supporters. We couldn't do it without all of you."

Because taking oxaliplatin is so devastating, Patrick got an occasional break from the drug. After he'd been on chemo for nearly a year, he wrote: "I strangely felt pride when Dr. Ng told me she had never seen anyone endure as many rounds with the oxaliplatin as I had: 24 rounds. Among the standard chemo side effects (nausea, fatigue, loss of appetite), this drug causes neuropathy. Neuropathy is a condition where the nerve endings in your hands and feet become destroyed. I remember working out at the gym and getting on the treadmill to do sprints. I was running, but I felt like I had no feet, they were completely numb and throbbing."

After he stopped taking the oxaliplatin, the neuropathy largely went away, except when he faced the cold. "When my hands/feet are exposed to any bit of cold now they turn numb, cramp up, and feel like I have a bunch of needles stabbing into them. Not fun. I keep begging Amanda to move down south to escape these winters... maybe one day."

Almost immediately after Patrick's diagnosis, I received a note from Peter Rabinowitz: "We are devastated to hear about Patrick; such a beautiful, loving, smart and joyous man. Our hearts go with you and the family, and we cheer him on! We are part of your team."

Through the early months of 2018, Peter's bone metastasis didn't respond to additional bone-directed therapies. The cancer overwhelmed his body. He became bed-bound and entered hospice care. I visited him in the Boston apartment where we had shared so many fond moments. A stack of books lay atop his nightstand and cable news channels were on the television. His voice was merely a whisper, his demeanor a far cry from the vivacious, self-assured, and colorful raconteur I had known. He had accepted that his death was imminent. He drifted off to sleep frequently during our conversation. After inquiring me how Kathy, Patrick and the other children were doing, he grasped my hand and asked if I would speak at his services. I said it would be my honor.

He died peacefully in his bed on May 27, 2018. Four days later, Kathy, Patrick, Kay, Brendan and I attended his service at Temple Israel in Boston. The front cover of the order of service booklet showed his picture and his signature statement: "Burn with a clear blue flame." Somehow, I was able to stay composed while speaking passionately about the dear friend I had made despite my initial misgivings about our compatibility.

From the time of Patrick's diagnosis, St. Luke's let me continue performing most of my job duties from my Massachusetts home. An occasional trip back to Idaho aside, I conducted my business chiefly through video conferences and conference calls. Meantime, I would join Patrick at Dana-Farber on most of his treatment days, and we would text or phone often. But it soon became imperative that I find a job much closer to home.

Patrick's employer, Northeast Security, let him continue working in a hybrid home-and-on-site arrangement, as best he could. The company—a multigenerational family-owned business—treated him in extraordinarily kind ways, suggesting that family values superseded the common practice of evaluating employees solely on productivity. It helped my son to stay tethered, to some extent, to the life he had known.

He also continued to work out. The activity not only connected him to a routine that had long been a regular part of his life, but medical evidence suggests that physical activity can lower the risk of getting cancer, and it's been shown that exercise is beneficial across the cancer-care continuum. Over time, Patrick also found some comfort by taking up yoga and meditation.

Though he hardly had an appetite, he put himself on a strict, healthy diet, eliminating processed foods, sweets and added sugars.

He continued to think somewhat regretfully about his time in the Marines. "I miss being in the Marines," he wrote in his private journal in January 2018. "I wish I had the chance to deploy and serve my country. I have this shame and guilt that I never did anything. It's hard to describe this feeling. I think only some feel it. I'm a smart, athletic man and I didn't serve my part like I could have.

"I just want to do something bigger than myself and make an impact. So many people just go through life like a robot just working jobs they don't really like or care about. Wearing that Marine uniform and becoming a Marine gave me more pride than anything else I've done. I've been thinking a lot lately about some of my memories and experiences in the Marines. I wish I had some more USMC discipline and pride earlier in my life."

He needed every particle of that discipline now as he endured the relentless treatment. He wrote in CaringBridge, "Despite the breaks and the halt of the oxaliplatin, we were caught in what seemed to be a never-ending cycle of a week of chemo and feeling like total trash, followed by a week of trying as best I could to detox, work out, and recover for the next round. But it got harder and harder. Not only physically, but mentally. The mental game has always been much worse. In the beginning, it was easy to be motivated to fight—the drugs were working and I wasn't feeling absolutely terrible most of the time.

"As time went on, it became harder and harder. It wears you down, every single day of your life. It consumes you. How do you continue to motivate yourself to go in and keep getting round after round for the rest of your life? That's what we were told: I would be on this chemo for the rest of my short life, hopefully extending my time by several months or (if lucky) a couple years."

Every three or four months, Patrick would get scans to track the effectiveness of his treatment. A scan on February 9, 2018, showed some promising news—most, if not all, of the lung nodules were smaller and no new ones had appeared. "A glimmer of hope," he wrote in his personal journal. "That's what this latest scan report has given me. Everything has continued to shrink, and the chemo is still working. Tomorrow is round # 9 and I have several questions for Dr. Ng. I'd like to know how much detectable cancer is left in my body. Maybe, just maybe, I can continue this treatment and it will lead me to a [no evidence of disease state]. But I can't get my hopes too high. Positive thinking. Take the good news when it comes.

"I'm 30 years old now. Crazy to think how fast time can go by. But I also feel like I've had cancer forever now and it's only been about 5 months… wish I could stop time in its tracks."

That same month, a national executive search firm reached out to me about a physician-executive opportunity at a health system on Long Island. In April, they made me an offer. While this new job couldn't match—in satisfaction and compensation—what I had in Boise, it met my major objective: to be much closer to home to support Patrick. In June, I started my new job on Long Island. I never revealed to my new employer the major reason why I took the job.

A real estate agent helped Kathy and me find a rental apartment in Huntington, on the north shore of Long Island, about 30 miles from my office in Garden City. But we kept our permanent residence in Medfield. On most Friday afternoons, I would be on a Cross Sound Ferry running from Orient Point to New London, Connecticut, followed by a 90-minute car ride home. Although the return trip would start very early on Monday mornings, I could spend weekends at home near my family.

When conditions at home allowed it, Kathy would spend a few days in Huntington. One day, browsing through local shops, she came upon a jewelry store, the Sedoni Gallery. A pair of cufflinks caught her attention. The cufflinks were adorned with the Superman icon of the bold "S"—a symbol for hope in the Superman story. Kathy told the salesperson, "I know a Superman. It's one of my sons. I'm going to get these for him."

A week later, while Patrick was seated in an infusion chair at Dana-Farber, she gave them to him, with a note: *"You are a Superman."*

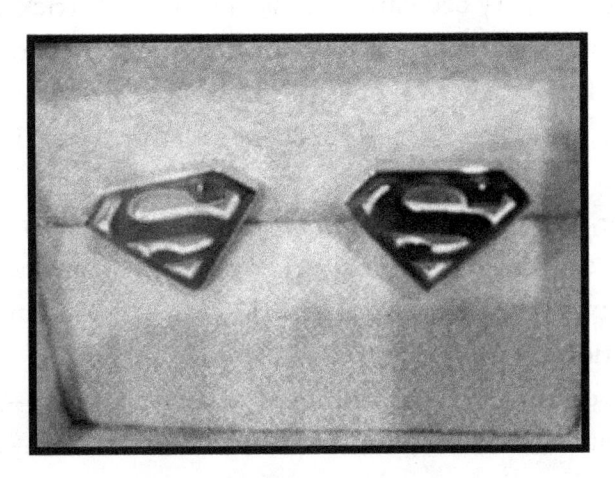

Photo Credit: Kathleen Beauregard

At the time of Patrick's diagnosis, nodules were present in both lungs, a spread extensive enough that surgically removing them would confer little to no survival benefit, as well as no reduction in the likelihood of recurrence. What's more, the surgery would take about 30 percent of Patrick's lungs, diminishing his functional status and quality of life, not to mention risking potential complications associated with the surgery itself.

By around June, after Patrick had been undergoing triplet chemotherapy and immunotherapy for about eight months, a CT scan of his chest showed further reductions in the number and size of the pulmonary nodules. That raised the possibility that surgery could remove any visible residual disease.

About that possibility, Patrick wrote, "If you are diagnosed with stage 4, pray that you are 'operable.' Meaning they can go in and surgically remove ALL (visible) cancer from your body. This is still by far your best option of being cancer-free. Not to say you are out of the woods then—many people still have the cancer return, typically it is only a matter of weeks, months or even years later. We kept pushing for possible lung surgery, but our doctor (and the tumor board at Dana-Farber) did not believe it would have any long-term benefits. So, was it even worth it?"

Still, with surgery becoming a possible option, Patrick and Amanda met with thoracic surgeons at both Brigham and Women's Faulkner Hospital and Tufts Medical Center to review a possible procedure. Later, Patrick wrote, "HOPE is the best medicine you can ask for in this. Then, everything changed."

Another scan in August 2018 revealed disastrous news: The cancer had progressed throughout the lungs. The nine or ten lung nodules spread through the two lungs had turned into 30-plus nodules. Surgery was no longer an option.

"We were a wreck," Patrick wrote. "It was tough timing—we received the news right before leaving for the weekend for one of my best friend's weddings, and I was in the wedding party. I could barely get myself to go. But I am so glad we did because it was a great escape to be surrounded by friends and we were distracted all weekend.

"The objective with stage 4 cancer (at least in the medical world) is that the cancer must be contained and stabilized for as long as possible. The worst news you can receive on a scan is that there are new locations found of the disease. Most common metastasis locations for colon cancer are the lungs and liver. Lucky for us, my liver has remained clear throughout this entirety. Many patients are diagnosed with metastases to both their liver and lungs, equivalent to getting two life sentences back-to-back. It's also very common for the cancer to spread throughout other areas of the abdomen, bones, and the brain. Cancer knows no boundaries—once it is in the bloodstream and lymphatic system it is free to float around wherever it pleases."

Patrick called to tell us about the scan results. As he delivered the dispiriting news, our hearts sank, but we did our best to listen and let him speak uninterrupted. Then we offered support in any way possible—a visit, food, anything. I asked him to share the report with me, which he later did.

Although I wasn't looking at the actual images, the words that described those insatiable, living mutations practically jumped off the page. In his stoic way, Patrick didn't like engaging in long telephone calls, especially ones involving bad news, so the conversation was brief. With his okay, we let his siblings know. Another pall hung over the family. But we knew we had to recharge quickly; whether or not Patrick could remained to be seen.

That August scan represented the first real setback Patrick had received since getting his stage 4 diagnosis. It hit Patrick hard—a real gut punch. But it wasn't a knockout punch. He got off the mat and refueled his determination to move forward in as positive a manner as he could. In a way, he was doing the Crucible again, the grueling Marine training exercise, and he knew he was capable of it. In his private journal, he wrote, "But what other option do you have besides to look ahead and press on? No reason to sit around wallowing in depression and pity, it will only make things worse. It's time for me to take a step back, take a deep breath and regroup. This too shall pass. Have faith, be grateful, and know that all this material and earthly bullshit means absolutely nothing in the end."

At the start of each day, Patrick now asked himself how he was going to better himself. And around this time, he and Amanda added a new member to the family—Ruby, a lively boxer puppy, whose antics served as welcome entertainment. Patrick particularly enjoyed taking her for walks and to the park.

The dreaded oxaliplatin and bevacizumab were resumed in his treatment cycles. He endured 8–12 rounds without a change in his regimen. Despite the obvious toll it was taking on him, his resilience persisted, motivating each of us to find creative, yet unobtrusive ways to support him and Amanda. Even taking Ruby on weekends became a tactic.

He later wrote: "It was utter hell. August 2018–February 2019 was perhaps the lowest of lows. I honestly don't know how Amanda managed to put up with me. Since the initial surgery and first few rounds of chemo, the scans showed that my abdomen was clear of cancer (at least visibly). While that was great, the lung nodules didn't improve during this time—they stayed stable at first, but then they became resistant and slowly started to grow along with the affected lymph nodes in my chest/neck region. What was the point of feeling half dead for exceptionally small results to show for it?"

Brendan had never been much of a runner, but that September he and Patrick decided to participate in the annual 5K Colon Cancer Coalition run ("Get Your Rear in Gear") held at Carson Beach in South Boston. The runs are held around the country to raise funds for cancer research.

Patrick had started to focus more time as a public advocate for colon cancer awareness, and the event's organizers asked him to speak to the runners and their families and friends before the run began. "If you're a patient, a survivor or caregiver," he told the crowd, "If you're still out there fighting like I am, know that you're not alone, so keep fighting and never give up."

Patrick couldn't run, but he walked the course. They were part of Team Panda, which included family and friends. Brendan took it as a warm-up for the Boston Marathon, which was to take place the following April.

As was customary for our family, Kathy and I hosted Thanksgiving and Christmas that year. Despite Patrick's condition, family dinners always ignited lively, often teasing conversation and laughter, as if, thank God, the pleasure we took in each other's company could overwhelm even the grimmest of news. For me, certainly, seeing all nine of us together—Kathy, me, our children, the two spouses and one soon-to-be spouse—brought immense joy, and I think that the entire extended family felt the same way.

As he progressed toward round 31 of chemo—with a couple of temporary reprieves from the oxaliplatin—Patrick enjoyed occasional dinners out with Amanda. A few weeks ahead of his 31st birthday on February 9th, we had a memorable family dinner at Del Frisco's Steakhouse, one of the best restaurants in Boston, and nestled in the Seaport District on historic Liberty Wharf. A bottle of fine wine was waiting for Patrick when he arrived, courtesy of an aunt and uncle. For that night, Patrick put aside his strict diet and mastered his lack of appetite enough to have a glass of wine, a seafood dinner, and a piece of Del Frisco's fabulous butter cake. It was a pleasure to watch.

# 10

# Reservations for Nine

ON A BUSY February afternoon in 2019, an email from my daughter appeared in my Inbox. Nothing was written in the "Subject" line, but a Word document titled "Reservations for Nine" was attached. I immediately sensed that this wasn't going to be about an actual reservation. I decided not to read it while at work and only opened it that evening.

*Reservations for Nine*

"A mid-September evening in 2017 was the last time my family lived unscripted. That night, reservations were made only for five, but this small party was no surprise as it was a weeknight. We were celebrating my birthday over mediocre margaritas and guacamole. Avocados are funny; one minute they're in perfect condition and the next they're quickly deteriorating. To compare my brother's health to the state of an avocado seems like an insensitive joke, however, this is how my sibling relationships have always been; we poke fun at each other, often disguising our insecurities with self-deprecating humor.

My brother Patrick wasn't with us that night, but I later learned that he had developed acute stomach pain with nausea and vomiting that necessitated a trip to the emergency room. During that ED visit, he was diagnosed with an intestinal obstruction. A CT scan of his abdomen, however, revealed that the joke was on us: Patrick had a mass in his colon. In that moment of diagnosis, it was as if all the laughter in the world was sucked right out. Rather than greeting each other with quick wit, we were all paralyzed in fear. That fear deepened when he subsequently learned that there was evidence that the cancer had already spread to his lungs; he had stage 4 disease, which current treatment options do not cure. Our family story changed from a romcom to a tragedy overnight, and my previously healthy 29-year-old brother was the unfortunate lead at the center of it all.

Without knowing how to move forward, we do. Appointments are made, oncologists are interviewed, scans are scheduled, and meal trains are full steam ahead. Meeting each other out for dinner was a time-honored, family pastime. Every meal shared together—at a fine steakhouse or seafood joint in the city or at our hometown staple—found the nine of us in sheer happiness. The same is true about a home cooked meal shared amongst each other, however, at this particular point, everything seemed so foreign, including eating meals prepared for us from loved ones. I know I loved Auntie Col's chicken piccata, but I just couldn't stomach it. Nobody could stomach Patrick's diagnosis.

In the same way diners wait between courses, we wait. We live in eight-week chunks, bi-weekly chemo followed by scans. More chemo, more scans. More waiting, more anxiety, more fear. Always more chemo. Four rounds of chemotherapy become 32. The latest scan shows that the cancer has progressed; the chemo is at a point where it is starting to fail. This pause in time is as expected and nerve wracking as the moment when the waiter comes to clear the main plates, asking if anyone is up for dessert. Does anyone feel up for cancer? No, we'll pass on cancer. You can bring us a clean bill of health instead.

My brothers and I had a childhood of dreams, with supportive parents who gave us everything we never knew we needed. The same is still true today, despite Patrick's cancer battle. My father, a veteran physician, does all he possibly can with his experience and knowledge to support Patrick and help him navigate the healthcare delivery system that is often a maze. My oldest brother believes in nothing but a cure, while my youngest brother remains committed to running the Boston Marathon to honor Patrick and raise thousands of dollars for cancer research. I find myself somewhere in between their two mindsets, depending on the day. Meanwhile, my mom has turned her kitchen upside down, replacing anything that's not organic. Her new vegan cooking goes well beyond the kitchen. These days, she is most often cooking up hope.

Our family, rooted in Catholic faith, has adopted the phrase "pray, hope, and don't worry," a nod to Padre Pio, a saint in the Roman Catholic Church. Shirts and sweatshirts adorned with that phrase are being worn by family and friends. Amidst all the life changes this past year-plus has tossed our way, we are all doing our best to face Patrick's diagnosis with the belief that we can all find happiness in the everyday. Of course, this is easier said than done. Some days it feels like we've all just come up empty and the numbing sensation feels permanent. But then we make reservations for nine and color rushes back to my cheeks; I'm invigorated and full of life at the thought of just being all together.

Sitting down to a table filled with family, it's easy to forget that you're there for the food. For our family, dining is all about savoring our time together. We share wine, we pass plates, we laugh at each other, and we cry with one another. My favorite moment when sitting down to dinner is when the table is abuzz with chatter, our family chatter, the most important buzz in all the restaurant. I always seem to find a moment to myself to take it all in, to look around at each and every one of us and relish the feeling of togetherness. The nine of us make up the most memorable table in the whole establishment, because it is our table, and we are all here together."

*The End*

Tears streamed down my face as I finished reading. In a paper submitted for a college creative-writing assignment, my daughter had captured the multiple feelings of our family.

Children are living miracles—somewhat like Belleek pottery pieces, each finely crafted and each with unique and delicate features. When a piece breaks, each porcelain shard must be recovered, and every attempt made to restore the pottery to a near-original, whole state.

# 11

# Team Panda Power

SOME 30,000 RUNNERS took part in the 123rd Boston Marathon on April 15, 2019. The day was early-spring cool and damp—around 54 degrees Fahrenheit and overcast following a heavy rain. Runner number 26734 was Brendan Beauregard, 20, a freshman at Emerson College. He ran as a team member of the Cam Neely Foundation for Cancer Care. Cam Neely, a former star power forward on the Boston Bruins hockey team and current president of the franchise, had lost both his parents to cancer. In their memory, he established the foundation, which raises funds to support cancer research and operates the Neely House, a bed-and-breakfast style home (located within Tufts Medical Center), for cancer patients undergoing treatment and their families. A month before, Patrick, Brendan, and I had toured the Neely House and briefly met Cam Neely himself during a Bruins game.

Brendan had encountered some doubts when he volunteered for the marathon team. Participating members are obligated to raise a minimum of $10,000 in donations, and the team's trainer and organizer worried about Brendan's ability to hit that mark, given his lack of running experience. Undaunted,

GEORGE BEAUREGARD

Brendan put up a fundraising page titled *Bbo4Pbo* that featured a picture of Patrick and him hamming it up together in an infusion room at Dana-Farber during Patrick's 22nd round of chemotherapy. Kathy and I were prepared to make up any shortfall beneath the $10,000 floor. That didn't prove to be necessary.

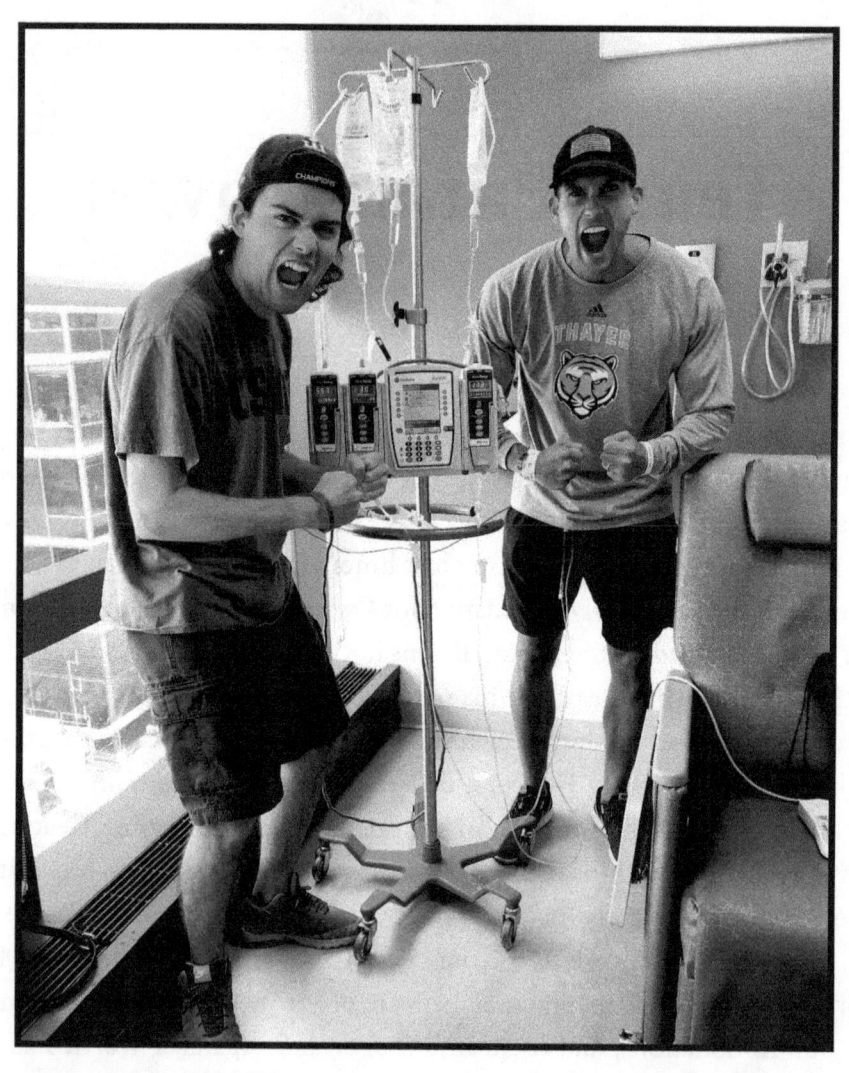

Photo Credit: Amanda Beauregard

Although he was in good physical shape and he'd run in a 5K race the fall before, Brendan was no marathoner. But he trained hard by running at home in the streets of Medfield and Boston, often wearing a blue-hooded sweatshirt with the words imprinted on the front, "In this family no one fights alone." On some days, Patrick joined him. "Here Pat was," Brendan recalled, "5:00 a.m. in the pitch dark, running in near single-digit temperatures alongside the water in South Boston only a few days after coming off the latest chemotherapy round."

Alerted by the head organizer of the marathon charity teams—who also had a connection to a local news outlet—some of the Boston media ran stories before the race about Brendan's endeavor. Explaining how he has managed the tough training, Brendan told WBZ, the Boston CBS TV station, Patrick is "trying to fight for his life, trying to live on, so it's what I want to do, and I just think about that whenever I hit a tough mile or a tough hill." To a reporter for the *Boston Herald*, Brendan said, "He's my hero in life."

By the day of the marathon, Brendan had raised slightly over $23,000 from more than 135 people.

Also running that day was Amanda's youngest sister, Devin, 25, another marathon novice, who ran as a member of the Dana-Farber charity team.

Brendan left the starting line at 11:15 a.m. and began the 26.2-mile grind to the finish line in downtown Boston. Underneath his official Boston Marathon race bib was a small, flat, oval-shaped silver medal given to him by his mother, who had received it from a close friend during the previous Christmas season. A single word was engraved on the medal: "Miracle."

Kathy and I positioned ourselves at the train depot in Framingham, 10 miles from the start and the first prime viewing spot. We watched our third son go by. His running gait was smooth and rhythmic, and he appeared focused and determined, bolstered by music on his Apple AirPods. The second good viewing spot, in Wellesley at around 17 miles, is called the Scream Tunnel, so named because during the first Boston Marathon in

1897 Wellesley students vociferously cheered on a Harvard runner. Kathy and I again watched Brendan churn past.

At mile 20 in Newton, runners encounter Heartbreak Hill, a steep, half-mile incline considered to be the hardest part of the course. As Brendan approached that obstacle, a familiar voice yelling encouragement broke through the music in his ears. His godmother, Mary Walsh, was waving her arms on the side of the route. He ran over and gave her a hug. She asked him how he was doing.

"Fine." And he was off again.

As the miles took their toll, Brendan later wrote, "Whenever I needed a boost, I thought of Pat and why we were doing this. Along with the fact that Pat himself would even join in on some of my training runs during treatment. That's always been an apt depiction of Pat for me whenever I talk about him. He simply did not let anything stop him from living his life the best he could. If he had that mentality, why couldn't any of us have it too in our own way?"

Running slowly on the eastbound side of Boylston Street, near Copley Square in downtown Boston, with his arms raised in a victory salute, Brendan crossed the finish line at 6:11:17 p.m. He kept going until a race worker told him his family was back near the finish line.

Patrick found him, and the two brothers walked side-by-side down Boylston Street, Patrick's left hand draped over Brendan's left shoulder. Brendan, covered by a foil blanket commonly given to marathoners who have completed the course, placed his right hand on Patrick's right upper arm. A photo of that moment sits atop my office desk.

RESERVATIONS FOR NINE

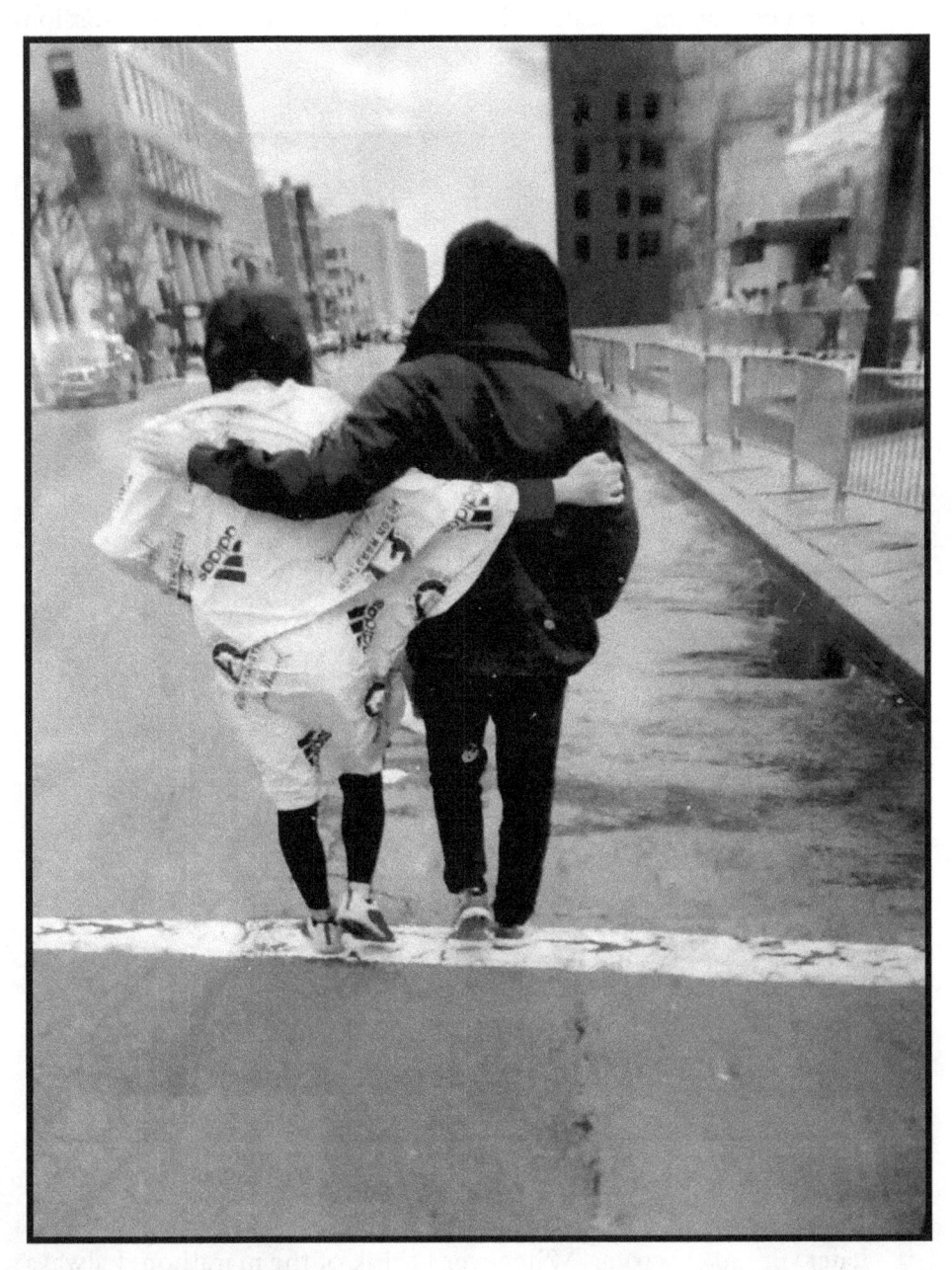

Photo Credit: Kim Neidermire

By the end of the day, donations had risen above $28,000. Mission Bbo4Pbo accomplished.

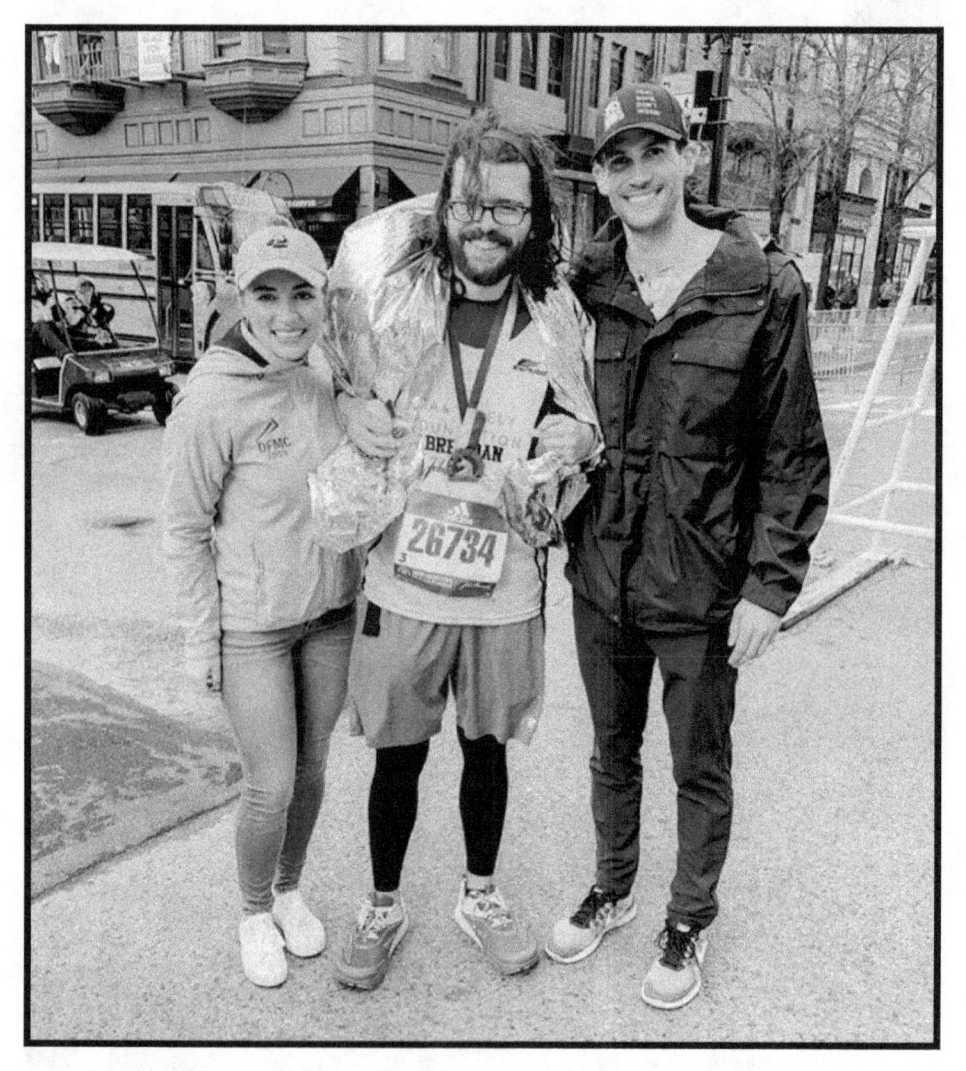

Photo Credit: Kim Neidermire

Later, Brendan wrote, "Whenever I think of the marathon, I always view it as Pat was the one running it, I was just the physical vessel for him that day. For months, I was logging in miles I never thought I would ever do. Some of those mornings were incredibly rough to run. As a first-time runner, I felt at times I was in over my head.

"I remember Marathon Monday itself as a near-complete blur. Crossing that famous blue and yellow finish line on Boylston Street is something I still cannot remember." He suspected that he blacked out. "What I do remember after is seeing my family and close friends, and walking with Pat." Of the photograph now cherished by his family, Brendan says, "For me, it symbolized one thing. That Pat, myself, and all of our supporters did what we set out to do that day. While it was nice and all to run, be featured on TV, and everything else, what truly mattered most from that time was sharing that accomplishment with my brother."

During an interview with the American Society of Clinical Oncology (ASCO) in April 2019, Patrick said, "Before my cancer diagnosis, I focused too much on the future and not enough on the present. I know it sounds counterintuitive, but, in many ways, cancer has changed my life for the better. I don't know what's ahead for me, I just know that for today, I'm living my best life."

Five months later, for the 2019 edition of the Colon Cancer Coalition run on September 14, at Carson Beach in South Boston, Team Panda Power sent about 90 people into the event. Brendan ran for the second year in a row. Others in the extended family accompanied him.

The year before, Patrick had walked the five-kilometer length of the race, but now he was in the throes of chemotherapy-induced fatigue. With me at his side, he slowly walked short distances along the route, periodically stopping to sit on benches to rest and catch his breath, greeting friends and shouting encouragement to the many runners and walkers passing in each direction.

While we walked, he couldn't talk much because of his shortness of breath, but we chatted loosely. In July, he had been honorably discharged from the Marines because of his medical condition, which he said was disheartening.

Our round trip probably covered somewhere between a quarter and half mile. Patrick admitted he felt lousy, but, notwithstanding, we drew solace from the experience. Still, I couldn't help noticing the blue posters placed at intervals along the route reading "In Memory of...." One poster read "In Honor of Patrick Beauregard" and featured a photo of Team Panda. I suppressed any thought of a sign saying, "In Memory of Patrick Beauregard."

Team Panda Power raised the highest level of donations that day for the local Colon Cancer Coalition.

# 12

# Looking for a Breakthrough

BY THE FALL of 2019, Patrick's determination to continue enduring chemotherapy was wearing thin. "After 33 rounds, it was becoming unbearable," he wrote in his CaringBridge blog. "I was a shell of what I was before I started chemo. Everyone would tell me I looked great, but I would look in the mirror and think I looked like death."

He recognized that the drugs that were devastating his body were no longer containing the cancer. "Over time, the cancer cells continue to adapt, evolve, and mutate, becoming invincible to the chemo drugs," he wrote. "Thankfully for us, the chemo was pretty effective at shrinking a lot of my cancer at first. Then it became stable. Then it started to grow very slowly. Once the effectiveness wore off, and the side effects became intolerable, we were finally presented with another option: a clinical trial."

Medical advances rely heavily on evidence from clinical trials. In their simplest form, clinical trials are research studies—involving human volunteers—designed to observe outcomes of the use of a drug or device under experimental conditions controlled by scientists. The official purpose is to *learn*—from successes and failures—not to treat patients, though researchers, of course, hope that their findings will lead to new treatments. Trials determine whether a new drug, device or treatment regimen is effective and safe. Although the length of a trial varies, the median completion time is about three years. Participation in a trial depends on meeting the patient eligibility criteria.

The first reported clinical trial dates to 1753—a Scottish naval surgeon experimented with treatments for scurvy and discovered that giving the afflicted sailors oranges and lemons worked. Ethical considerations weren't introduced until the mid-20th Century, after the infamous Tuskegee syphilis experiment was exposed to the public—the course of the disease in 399 African American men was observed but not treated. The news prompted outrage and new federal laws and regulations requiring institutional review boards. Even with careful regulation, a flawed clinical trial can pose risks and even inadvertently harm patients.

Grants from the National Institutes of Health fund most basic research in academic laboratories. However, about 75 percent of the funding for clinical trials comes from corporate sponsors, such as pharmaceutical companies (often called Big Pharma). These companies have enormous financial stakes in the products being evaluated. Although industry sponsorship of clinical trials can lead to important therapeutic advances, the potential exists for conflicts of interest and biased study results.

Trials are classified as phases. Phases I and II assess drug safety and potential efficacy. The knowledge gained from those phases inform Phase III trials. Those involve a larger and more diverse subject population and determine effectiveness as well as the incidence of common adverse reactions. The most common type of Phase III trials are "comparative efficacy" trials—one patient population gets the treatment being tested while a similar population gets a placebo or the standard pre-existing therapy.

Trials need to show evidence of causal—not corollary—effect. That is, it must clearly demonstrate that the tested treatment directly affected the infirmity. Randomized controlled trials (RCTs) are the study design of choice for drawing inferences about the association between treatment and patient outcomes. In those trials, qualifying participants are randomly assigned to either the group receiving the tested treatment or the one getting a placebo or "usual care." Even with well-designed and rigorously conducted clinical trials, it's tough to figure out how well the results of a clinical trial will translate to the real world. Historically, the adoption of medical evidence into clinical practice varies widely based on a range of factors. One notable analysis published in 2011 showed that it takes an average of 17 years for evidence to change practice widely. In my own practice, I repeatedly asked myself whether the trial findings applied to my individual patients and whether the results were strong enough to change to the new drug, treatment protocol or device.

Over the years, numerous clinical trials have significantly affected the practice of modern medicine. For example, in the so-called MERIT-HF study, conducted in 1997–98, an international team of researchers found that drugs known as beta-blockers substantially improved outcomes in patients with serious heart disease. The Women's Health Initiative study, sponsored by the National Heart, Lung and Blood Institute and published in 2002, demonstrated that combination hormone replacement therapy for menopausal women was associated with significant increases in heart disease, blood clots and breast cancer. (Subsequent analyses revealed, however, that, with adjusted confidence intervals, the heart disease and breast cancer risks were not statistically significant).

In any event, medical knowledge has been expanding exponentially. In 1950, it doubled every 50 years. By 2011, according to a study published in *Nature*, such knowledge was doubling every 3.5 years. (Estimates made then suggested that by 2020 medical knowledge would double every 73 days). Another study, published in the journal *Public Library of Science* in

2019, found that about 7,300 publications of clinical trial results appeared in four major national and international medical databases annually. It begs the question: How's a practicing doctor supposed to keep up with developments in his or her specialty amidst this ever-rising flood of new information?

As Patrick's disease progressed, he began hoping to participate in a clinical trial. With a doctor father and in the care of Dr. Ng, he was well situated to explore possibilities. But his independent and inquisitive nature also eased his way. As a child and into adulthood, Patrick rarely accepted assertions at face value. He was always one to ask "Why?" to the first statement and then to the answer as well. (As a parent, I sometimes found this quite annoying—in part because it reflected my own approach).

On many occasions over the years, Patrick had observed how I responded to people seeking advice from me about something medical they had read or seen on the Internet. Almost always, my response was simply: "What was the source of the information? Was it from a reputable publication or something else?" True to his nature, Patrick didn't idly sit by and wait for information to come to him as he fought his cancer. Over time, he became adept at confining his medical searches to reliable, scientific sources. He occasionally surprised me by passing on posts from Twitter or other widely used social media from people citing such scientific journals as *Nature* and *The New England Journal of Medicine*.

He also started searching out clinical trials by scouring reputable sources. These included the National Institutes of Health's ClinicalTrials.gov database and other clinical-trial listings with state and federal agencies, the American Cancer Society, and such private-sector research institutions as the Mayo Clinic, Cleveland Clinic, Johns Hopkins University, and European research centers and patient advocacy groups. He often sent me information about trials related to stage 4 colorectal cancer that were impending or currently accepting new patients. Occasionally, he shared abstracts from articles published in reputable journals for me to review. Sometimes, we would have conversations that led to questions to pose to Dr. Ng. (I never reached out to her without his approval).

As I said, Patrick was particularly well situated to search out clinical trials. Surveys have shown that most patients without his advantages turn to the news, to search engines and websites and even to social media for knowledge about research and evidence-based medicine. (A surprising number of people are skeptical about medical research). Statistics don't tell us how clinical trial participants learned of the trials, but only about 8 percent of cancer patients participate. The low rate can have to do with many factors—lack of information, fear of randomization into a particular arm, apprehension about side effects, and logistical challenges related to getting to distant academic medical centers.

Many of the clinical trials Patrick researched didn't have openings for new participants. Others did but had eligibility criteria that excluded him from consideration. In many of them, prolonging survival was the desired primary outcome—not cure. That notwithstanding, Patrick always remained hopeful that a trial might produce results far beyond that objective. I knew that, at best, trials offered a remote chance of extending his survival for more than a matter of months. But I didn't want to dampen any hope that Patrick had while combating his illness. He just had to hang on long enough until a breakthrough treatment became available.

In June 2018, Patrick and Amanda flew to San Francisco to attend the Cancer Research Institute's Immunotherapy Patient Summit and met with a clinical trial navigator to help Patrick find trials for which he might be eligible. Nothing seemed right. Then, in November 2018, he and Amanda traveled to HonorHealth—a non-profit hospital system based in Phoenix that has a cancer-care network and research services. They met there with a specialist in clinical trials.

Patrick later wrote, "While we were excited to hear about the different clinical trials that were ongoing/in the works at HonorHealth, ultimately, we decided that the best course of action at the time was to stick with the standard chemotherapy protocol. None of the available trials seemed like a great fit and we wanted to ride it out as long as we could and give the doctors and researchers time to refine and improve the trial treatments."

One of the promising areas of research focused on immunotherapy—treatments that help the patient's immune system fight the cancer. Since the early 2000s, research has explored the combination of immunotherapy and chemotherapy for treating certain cancers. Already, Patrick had been taking one immunotherapy drug, Avastin, but the nature of his cancer had so far precluded others.

Immunotherapy can take a variety of forms. Tumors exist in a complex ecosystem, and the factors that influence their growth and response to therapy are highly dynamic and complex. But researchers have given close attention to immune checkpoints—molecules that regulate the immune system's response, so it doesn't get over-active and damage healthy tissues. But these checkpoints also make it easier for cancer cells to evade the immune response. Twenty or so years ago, researchers developed drugs known as immune checkpoint inhibitors that specifically limit the proteins that dampen the immune response. In other words, these drugs unleash the immune system to go full throttle against the cancer. (Of course, that also means that the immune system is freer to overreact to healthy cells). In 2014, the U.S. Food and Drug Administration (FDA) approved two checkpoint inhibitors, opening the door for use of these therapies in various cancers. The introduction and use of these drugs—a major advance in treating patients with cancer—has moved beyond palliative care for patients with lung cancer and melanoma and now extends survival among patients with several forms of cancers, including lung, bladder and certain types of colorectal cancer. (Recent research even suggests that combining immunotherapy—checkpoint inhibitors—and radiotherapy may enhance the local and distant antitumor response, the so-called abscopal effect, from the Latin root words meaning "far" and "target").

In early 2019, Kimmie Ng alerted Patrick to a clinical trial at Dana-Farber that involved an immunotherapy drug that might be effective despite the nature of his tumors. He applied and was accepted. By then, he had endured 33 rounds of FOLFOXIRI and Avastin. In preparation for the trial, he got off the chemotherapy for a two-month wash-out period, and in April 2019, started the new regimen. (On this trial and others in which he participated, he always knew he was getting the experimental drug, not a placebo). The trial's objective was to investigate the effectiveness of a combination of two drug types: One was a checkpoint inhibitor (brand name Tecentriq) specifically targeted to block a protein found on the surface of some cancer cells; the second was the oral form of 5-FU (brand name Xeloda), which Patrick referred to as "the little pink nasties." He tolerated the therapy for three months, but his cancer progressed, and he withdrew from the trial.

"While you may see triumphant stories in the news of people receiving immunotherapy and their cancer just shrinking away, that happens in very few patients," he wrote in a CaringBridge entry. "Especially so with this type of cancer. Only about 30% of ALL cancer patients benefit even just SLIGHTLY from immunotherapy, let alone be cured from it. We knew it would be a long shot of it being effective for us. Despite feeling so good on the trial (very few side effects), it had no effect on the cancer. Blood work in June suggested that the cancer was continuing to grow, and we made the decision to get off the trial. It wasn't easy, I was just starting to feel somewhat 'normal' again. My appetite was back, I was gaining some weight, and was finally able to get back into a solid routine at the gym and at work. And now we had to change it all.

"I can't speak for Amanda or others, but getting kicked off the trial made me feel hopeless. I refused to give up, but I felt like we were presented with zero good options moving forward—we could go back to the chemo regimen I had been doing all along, but it may now essentially be ineffective, and my doctor was hesitant that my body would be able to withstand any more punishment."

Patrick rarely mentioned his more despairing thoughts to Kathy and me—for the most part, he left them for his personal journal. But as his prospects declined, he went from May 2019 to March 2020, without making any entries.

Patrick and Amanda had been planning a trip to France for over a year, and because he was feeling physically better from being off the chemo, he and Amanda decided to go. France had always had a special place in the hearts of our family. When she was a sophomore in high school, Kathy took a memorable trip to Paris, where her rakish Uncle Scotty had attended the Sorbonne and whose tales of French adventures intrigued her and later our kids. In June 2016, I surprised Kathy by buying tickets to one of Adele's world tour concerts held at the Accor Arena in Paris. Kathy and I spent nearly a week in Paris, visiting the Louvre Museum, Notre Dame Cathedral and other landmark sites.

For me, any trip to France had to include a visit to Normandy—the sacred place where a crucial turning point in World War II led to the liberation of Western Europe from the death grip of the Nazis. Kathy was initially reluctant to go, as she felt she might not be able to handle "being at a place where thousands of young people died." But together we viewed Omaha Beach and other landing spots. The American Cemetery and Memorial was somber, but beautiful. I viewed it with reverence. Normandy was the most memorable and overwhelming part of our trip. Before Patrick and Amanda left for France, he told me that what he most wanted to experience was Normandy.

After visiting Paris and the Loire Valley, they did just that. "Just got back from an all-day Normandy tour," Patrick later wrote. "Absolutely incredible. Should be a mandatory visit for all the sissies of today to see how good they really have it, thanks to those brave men."

He was also awed by Mont-Saint-Michel, the castle-like abbey on a tiny island just off the Normandy coast. "Probably the most breathtaking and awe-inspiring place I've ever experienced. Just incredible, pictures do not even show a fraction of its beauty."

RESERVATIONS FOR NINE

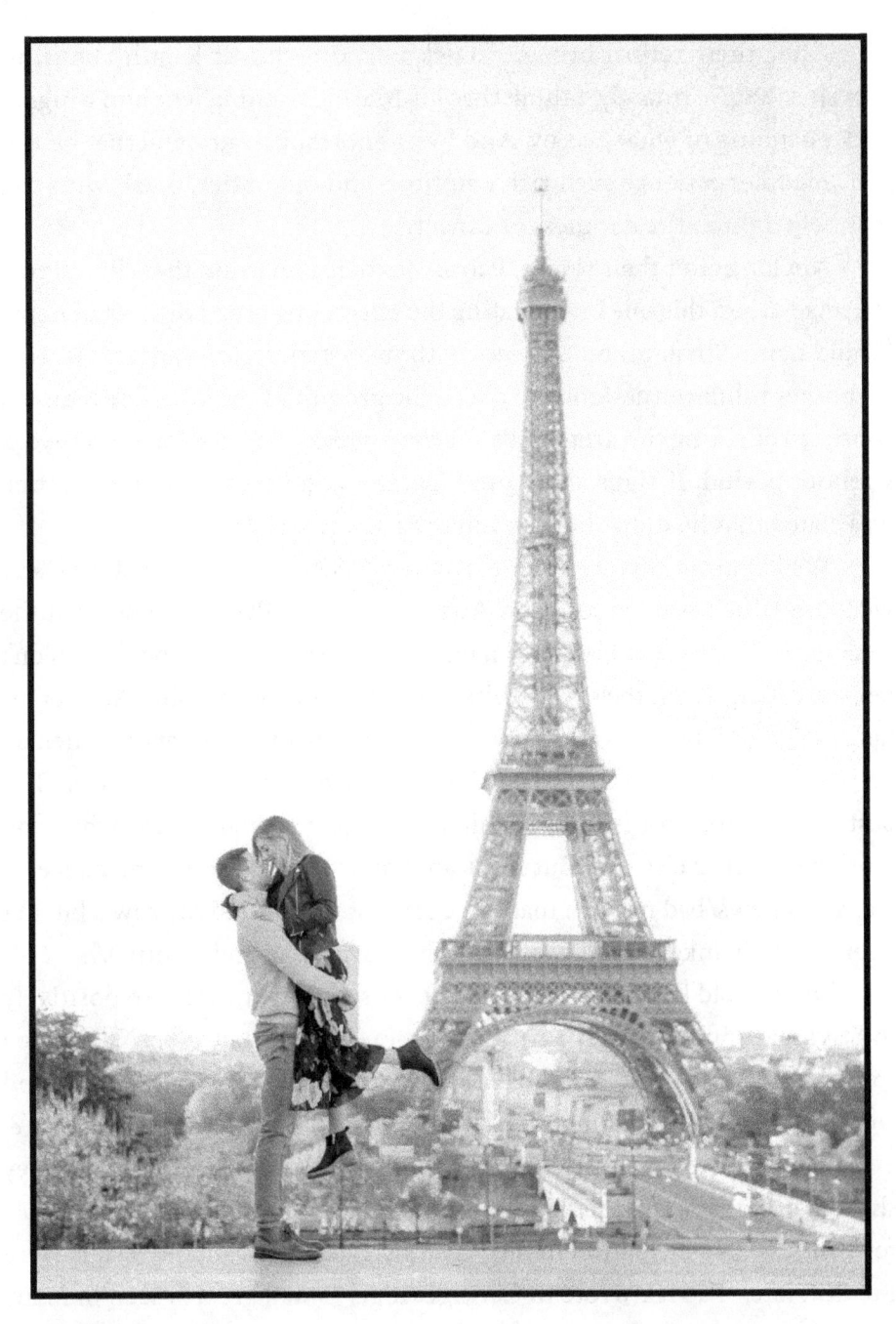

Photo Credit: Daniel Cojocaru

After their return home, Patrick talked to me at length about his experience at Normandy. I think that his Marine training lent him a higher understanding of what he saw. And I was enormously grateful that he was still able to experience such rich emotions and memories. Small wins like that help lighten the darkness of cancer.

Not long after their return, Patrick participated in another clinical trial at Dana Farber, this one investigating the effects of a drug called regorafenib (brand name Stivarga) on patients with metastatic colon cancer. Stivarga is another inhibitor designed to check the growth of tumors. The regimen consisted of taking the drug orally for three weeks, followed by a one-week washout period. If signs show promise, the regimen is repeated. Patrick was elated that he didn't have to undergo any infusions.

While on the Stivarga regimen, Patrick had a scan right before Dan's wedding which was to occur on August 30, 2019. Pat later described the wedding as "an absolute blast and an unforgettable experience," but he couldn't help worrying about the scan results. Happily, they showed shrinkage of his lung nodules. "Stivarga is a last-resort option for many colon cancer patients," he wrote. "It is never meant to cure, let alone even shrink your cancer. The best you can hope for is some stability for a short period of time while you work something else out. But my scan results showed some shrinkage! It was good news/bad news in that some areas still appeared to grow a bit, but overall the shrinkage seen was incredibly surprising and positive."

Dr. Ng told Patrick that she had never seen anyone react so positively to Stivarga alone. Given the better-than-expected results, Dr. Ng decided to add Xeloda, the oral 5-FU drug that Patrick had previously taken and continue the Stivarga regimen. The next scan was scheduled for November 8.

Patrick was optimistic, but the scan results were troubling. They showed progression in the size of his nodules, thus rendering him ineligible for continued participation in the Stivarga trial. "All in all, the results were not horrible," Patrick wrote in CaringBridge. "Small growth seen in many of the lung nodules, but no new spots or signs of disease (always a HUGE win). Containment is #1 priority. Then you can focus on taking care of the rest. The biggest pain in the ass with all of this is finding a new treatment. It sucks to have to transition to something new; so many appointments, visits, information, tests that get thrown at you so quickly and completely disrupts your life right when you start to relax a bit and get in a groove. The more options we run through, the less (and more inferior) options we have in front of us."

Still, Patrick pressed forward with his usual determination. "BUT we are moving onward and upward as always. What else can you do? I am still just happy at still being alive, to be honest. Every day is a gift. And we still have all the hope, motivation, and fight in the world left in us. This will not discourage us one bit." He said he was reaching out to other cancer centers around the U.S. "to see what else may be out there."

Meantime, another potential concern floated up. Patrick had been undergoing scans about every two to three months to monitor his response to treatments. The CT scans rely on radiation, which can cause harm, though on a lower scale than chemo drugs.

Radiation exposure is measured in millisieverts (mSV). On average, people reach exposure from natural sources of about 2 to 3 mSV each year. The radiation dose from a chest CT scan ranges from 5 to 10 mSV. Given the number of scans Patrick had during the initial 24 months of his treatment, he'd likely been exposed to anywhere between 60 and 150 mSV. Although well below the whole-body threshold where symptoms and potentially life-threatening effects can occur, there is no clear threshold below which no biological damage occurs. Accordingly, safety guidelines and protocols exist to minimize unnecessary exposure and ensure that the benefits of the procedure outweigh the risks.

As I thought of this, and the vulnerability of reproductive cells, I was glad that Patrick had banked his sperm before starting his treatments.

Throughout Patrick's ordeal, I wanted to leverage my experiences as a physician to help him however I could. Still, it saddened me that over many months, most text messages between us resembled a conversation between a doctor in training and an established physician, rather than the normal discourse between a father and son. I hoped that we'd be able to return to the latter before long.

But on another front, we had an intimate connection that became a small treasure in its own way. One of the surveillance CT scans of Patrick's chest revealed that he had a pulmonary embolism—a blood clot in one of the major vessels of his lungs. Although he had no symptoms typically associated with blood clots of that sort—primarily sudden chest pain and shortness of breath—the discovery was concerning. Cancer is a known risk factor for blood clots. So Patrick had to take an oral anticoagulant. He was started on apixaban, commonly known as Eliquis.

Coincidentally, I'd been on Eliquis for years for my atrial fibrillation. Some 30 years apart in age, my son and I were on identical medications. It came in handy when one of us was out of the drug and awaiting a prescription refill. Eliquis needs to be taken twice daily. Patrick, in his usual, disciplined manner, never missed a dosage. Every so often, I would forget to take the second dose. With a smirk, Patrick enjoyed reminding me to take the evening dose. Yet another small connection that came as a blessing.

# 13

# Brothers

THOUGH SEPARATED IN age by more than a decade, Patrick and Brendan had always been particularly close. Dan was also part of the brothers' team, but from the time of Brendan's birth, Patrick showed a special attachment to his younger brother.

They shared some physical traits. Both were left-handed (estimates are that only 10–15% of people are left-hand dominant), and both fell into the higher growth percentiles. Later on, like Patrick, Brendan immersed himself in video games, and, like Patrick, occasionally displayed a sardonic sense of humor. Patrick enjoyed mentoring his younger brother and always welcomed having him around. After Brendan enrolled at Emerson College in Boston, he often got together with Amanda and Patrick, sometimes staying overnight in their South Boston apartment. Over the years, watching the growing bond between Patrick and Brendan delighted Kathy and me.

Brendan later described their connection: "My relationship with Pat can best be called what our Dad used to refer to us as: 'thing one and thing two'—the human-like twins from Dr. Seuss's *The Cat in the Hat* book. I was actually trying to be like Pat. Pat was full of wit, determination, strength, and humility—attributes anyone would want to emulate. Though we were 11 years apart, the age gap meant nothing. He was my best friend, mentor, and my hero."

In November 2019, a scan revealed the possibility that Patrick's cancer had spread to his liver. "For the first time in a long time, I had radio silence from [Pat]," Brendan recalled. "We talked every day, and after not hearing from him for almost 36 hours, I felt helpless. I couldn't imagine what was running through his mind."

Patrick needed a respite, however brief, from his battle. (Because of his condition, doctors didn't address the liver issue at that point). Fortunately, through a Facebook cancer support group, he'd learned about a cottage in rural Georgia that was available free as a retreat for people with cancer. Founded by a breast cancer survivor, "Second Wind Cancer Retreat" sits in a woody, hilly and picturesque area near the Tennessee border. It offers, as its website says, "a peaceful place where people dealing with cancer can get away from the stresses of treatment for a few days, relax in a beautiful environment and gain new strength, energy and momentum." Patrick arranged a brief stay. He asked Brendan, then a sophomore at Emerson, to join him.

A couple of weeks before they were scheduled to leave, the brothers were invited by the Cam Neely Foundation for Cancer Care to attend an event in Boston. Prior to going to the event, they made plans to meet for dinner at Bencotto, an Italian restaurant in Boston's North End. Earlier that day, an email popped up in Brendan's mailbox.

"I have [been] struggling for a while now to put the thoughts in my head into text," Patrick wrote Brendan. "There has been so much going on lately that, at times, it can feel a bit overwhelming. The physical side effects and issues with chemo and cancer treatment [are] well known. What is often less discussed is the mental side of things. And, for me, this is much more difficult.

"I have struggled mightily lately. So much so that I have decided it best for me to reach out for help to speak with someone. I will see a therapist at Dana-Farber soon. This disease is hell. It consumes every minute of your life. My entire existence is based around me trying to survive and beat this thing. As the months drag on, the longer and harder the fight becomes. A war of attrition indeed. This disease is so good at chipping away at your confidence, your hope, your motivation, every single chance it can get. At times, I wonder what is left inside me after being stripped of so much.

"Yet sometimes all it takes is the smallest of things to recenter your focus and re-arm your motivation. This exact thing happened to me just the other day—here's the story:

"I was cleaning out my drawers and trying to organize a bunch of items, files, etc. I was in a foul mood. I didn't feel well, I didn't feel like dealing with anyone or work or anything. I just wanted to be left alone; I was exhausted with barely an inch of fight left inside of me. And then, I found a note inside my drawer which I had folded in half. It was a small piece of paper and I thought perhaps it might be some work notes from a meeting I had or something. It turned out to be something much different. A tiny note with just 11 words written on it that entirely changed my mood and recharged my fight.

"It was your note you left me one-time last winter when I was on chemo. The note reads: '3:10 pm.... Left for the train. Didn't want to wake you. Keep battling brother.—B

"I immediately broke down in tears. It's amazing what the human brain is capable of because a rush of emotions came over me immediately. Flashbacks of everything we have endured and gone through these past 2+ years, the longest years of my life. It reminded me how far we have come and how different things are now. You are correct, there is much work left to do, and my only goal in life is to help as many as I can who are out there struggling much worse than I ever could imagine. But first, time to once and for all beat the shit out of this beast inside of me. I sent you that article about how some cancer patients do not like being referred to as 'warriors' or 'battlers fighting a war.' Well I thought more on that and I disagree. I am a military man. I was trained for battle. I relish the fight. I meditate often and imagine myself and my army of supporters behind me crushing the cancer cells in my body.

"I must go on. I have too many people relying on me, it's not just about me." He had just helped to raise a substantial sum for colorectal cancer research. "It's a lot," he continued. "More money than I've ever seen at one time in my life. It's helpful, but that's not what matters. What matters is what we do with our time here. And I fully intend on using [it] to bring as much good into the world as possible and help as many as I can.

"I am excited for tonight, and especially for next weekend. I think you will have a lot of fun hiking and being out in the woods. It's so peaceful and beautiful.

"I love you brother. I am so damn proud of the man you are. You've honestly been my #1 supporter throughout this, and it means the world to me. You are my hero too, I hope you always know that.

"P.S. I have some big news for you tonight. See you soon."

After Brendan and Patrick had settled at their table in the lively Italian restaurant, Patrick disclosed the big news. "I still remember everything from that night," Brendan later wrote. "Pat's ear-to-ear smile as he said, 'Amanda is pregnant.'

"To hear Pat's joy of becoming a father, his resolve to keep living his life and not let cancer control it, I cherish that moment and wish I could be back there that night. Along with reliving the exact time I received the email he sent earlier that day."

The brothers flew down to Atlanta and rented a Dodge minivan for the two-hour drive to the cottage, stopping along the way to pick up groceries. The cottage, near a horse farm, was rustic but lovely and isolated—no Wi-Fi, limited cell phone service, a DVD player and old box TV on which they watched a scratchy copy of *Almost Famous* the first night. A comfortable front porch offered rocking chairs. "In many ways, that place gave us a second wind," Brendan said.

Brendan was dismayed to learn Patrick was down to 160 or so pounds. "Pat had always been a tall and muscular guy, always around 200 pounds—having the physique of those you see in superhero movies like Henry Cavill's Superman or Chris Hemsworth's Thor. Now he was around the same weight I was and dropping. It was not right."

Still, one day, the brothers took a round-trip 8.5-mile hike along the Toccoa River, and Patrick managed despite his increasing frailty. "During those couple of hours, we talked about a lot of things," Brendan recalls. "Life, death, our fears, everything. I still can hear Pat talk about being afraid of not being around for his unborn child, Amanda, and the whole family, but still just wanting to live today and move forward as best we can. The wisdom Pat wielded was always insurmountable."

As fans of history, Patrick and Brendan drove to Fort Oglethorpe, Georgia, the site of the bloody Civil War battle known as Chickamauga. They visited a museum and the battlefield grounds, where Brendan savored tapping his brother's "Marine intellect."

One night at a local diner, they ordered a platter of fried pickles. "I can still hear Pat's laugh and him saying, "Haven't had this in forever," Brendan recalled. "Small moments like that made the trip special."

GEORGE BEAUREGARD

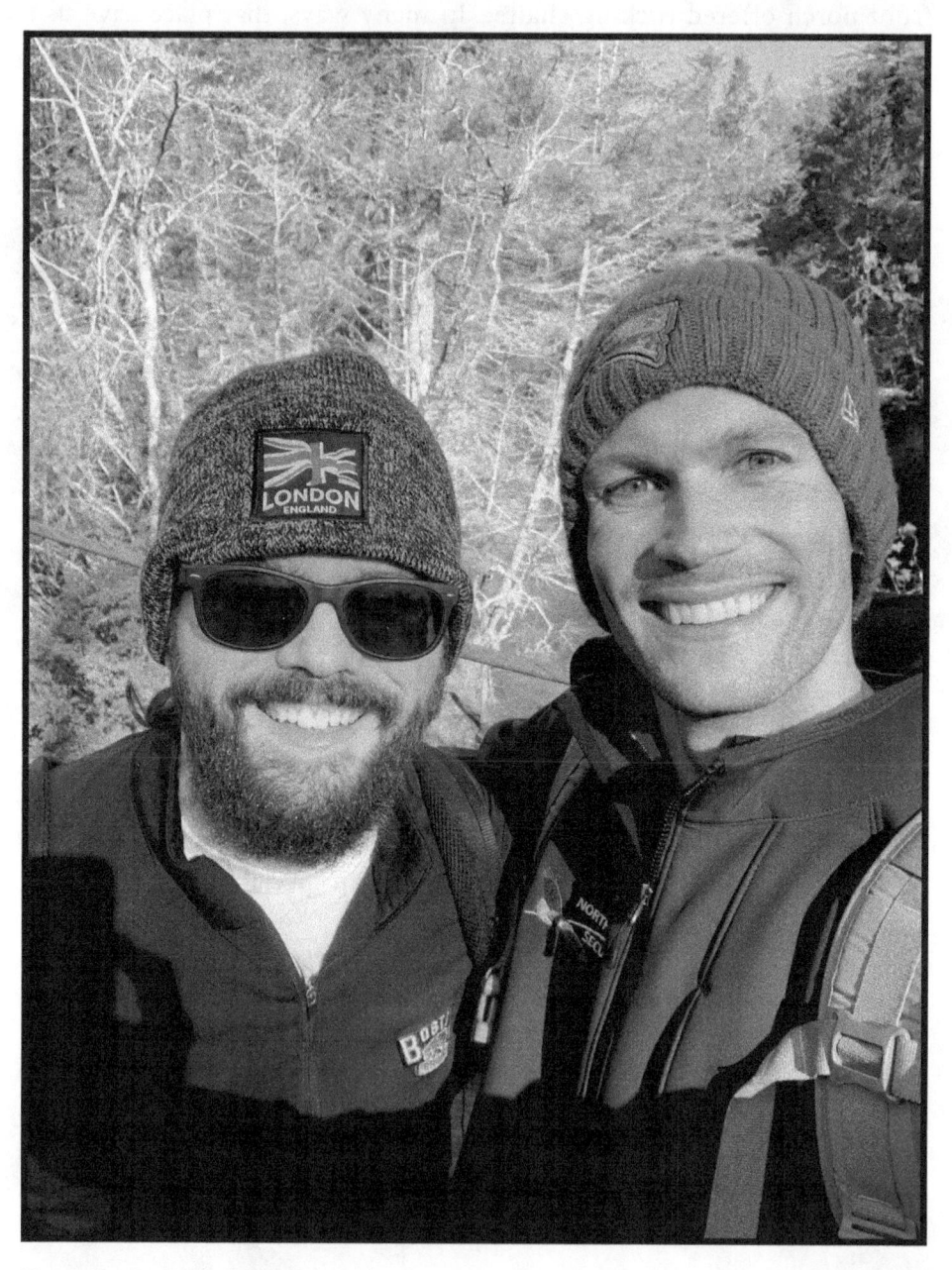

Photo Credit: Patrick Beauregard

The brief retreat came as a welcome break for both brothers. "It was just what I needed to clear the head and recharge for the fight ahead," Patrick said. Brendan later wrote, "Georgia was such an important time for Pat and me. It gave us new life in our own ways." They didn't know what was coming in the following months, but they both felt vastly better after the trip.

Brendan continued to reflect on the words of Patrick's email the day of their dinner at Bencotto. "There is no greater honor I could receive that will top Patrick calling me his hero, too," Brendan wrote. "They are words I try my best to live up to."

# 14

# Glimmers of Hope

WHEN PATRICK'S DIAGNOSIS came back as stage 4 colon cancer, I knew there was no therapy to cure him, and I knew the grim survival-rate numbers. The KRAS mutation in his tumors made the situation even more dismal. But with medical advances occurring regularly, I wanted him to hang on long enough for the possibility of a breakthrough.

The year after Patrick's diagnosis, a medical journal reported that one new treatment involving a form of immunotherapy showed promise against some solid tumors. I let myself hope that this might be the breakthrough that Patrick needed.

This new treatment—known generally under the name adoptive cellular therapy—is a form of immunotherapy that improves the cancer-fighting ability of cells from the body's immune system. Basically, here's how it works: The immune system contains so-called tumor-infiltrating lymphocytes (TILs), naturally occurring white blood cells that attack and discharge toxic chemicals into cancer cells. While many patients do mount a spontaneous immune response to cancer cells, the effectiveness is blunted by mechanisms produced by the cancer cells that can deactivate or diminish the immune response. Over time, scientists discovered that they could enhance the strength of the TILs by re-engineering them outside the patient's body, then re-injecting them to go after the cancer with new capabilities and vigor.

Specifically, the treatment takes T cells—the cancer fighter in the TILs—and boosts them by adding more Chimeric Antigen Receptors, which let T cells recognize markers on the cancer cell surface and after binding to it, steer in killing capabilities.

The system is called CAR-T therapy. Initially developed in the late 1980s and early 1990s, the clinical application of CAR-T started gaining attention in the 2010s. The FDA approved it in 2017 for use in pediatric and young adult patients with a specific kind of leukemia, and the results have been promising. Now, scientists are experimenting with using the therapy on other cancers, including colon cancer.

During October 2019, while on Stivarga and Xeloda, Patrick reached out to the National Institutes of Health (NIH) in Bethesda, Maryland, expressing his interest in being considered for a TILs trial NIH was running. Because he was on treatment at the time, he was ineligible to participate. But when scans showed that the disease was spreading, his doctors discontinued the regimen. The oncology team at Dana-Farber recommended that he consider participating in another Dana-Farber trial, but Patrick wanted to explore other options. He knew of the TILs research, and he and I had several conversations about the science behind this new therapy. I strongly encouraged him to try to participate in the NIH trial.

He again approached NIH, and he was invited for screening. After visiting the NIH and going through a flurry of tests, in December he was officially accepted. The process would begin in January—he would return to NIH for surgery to harvest the tumor cells to start the procedure. I tempered my excitement so as not to give Patrick or the rest of my family false hope—this therapy was in its infancy for solid tumors such as colon cancer. But if there was going to be a miracle–which my son desperately needed–this might be it. A stronger sense of renewed hope stirred deep within me.

That made for a welcome spot of cheer for Christmas that year. More cheer would soon follow. For many years, Kathy and I hosted immediate and extended family members for Christmas Day gatherings. Patrick and Amanda spent Christmas Eve with the Floods and arrived at our house mid-morning on the 25th. When it was time to exchange gifts, they presented a nicely wrapped box to Kathy and me.

Inside the box was a Christmas tree ornament, a round white ceramic disk. The front displayed an announcement: **BABY BEAUREGARD, Coming July 2020.** The back carried an ultrasound image of a small fetus. This was the first time that we'd heard that Amanda was pregnant! Brendan had kept the secret. Amanda had undergone the In-vitro fertilization process at Massachusetts General Hospital several months earlier. (It would be another month before we learned that their baby would be a boy.)

GEORGE BEAUREGARD

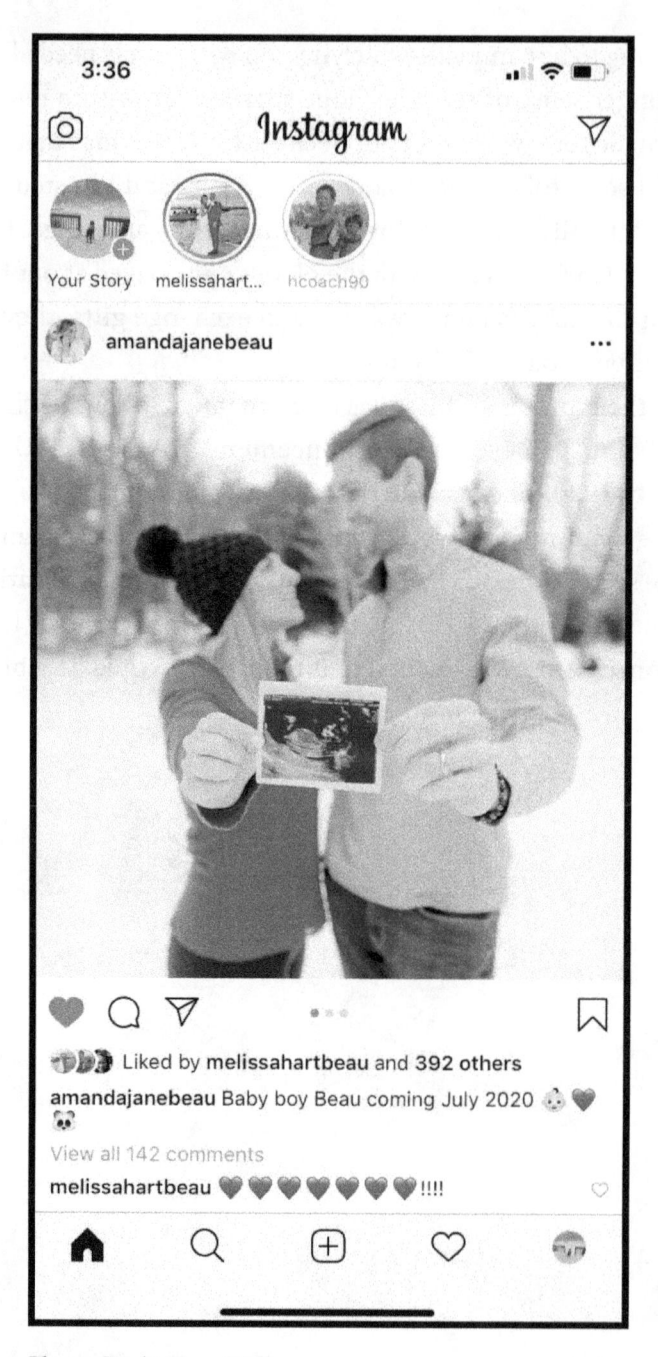

Photo Credit: Jane Miller

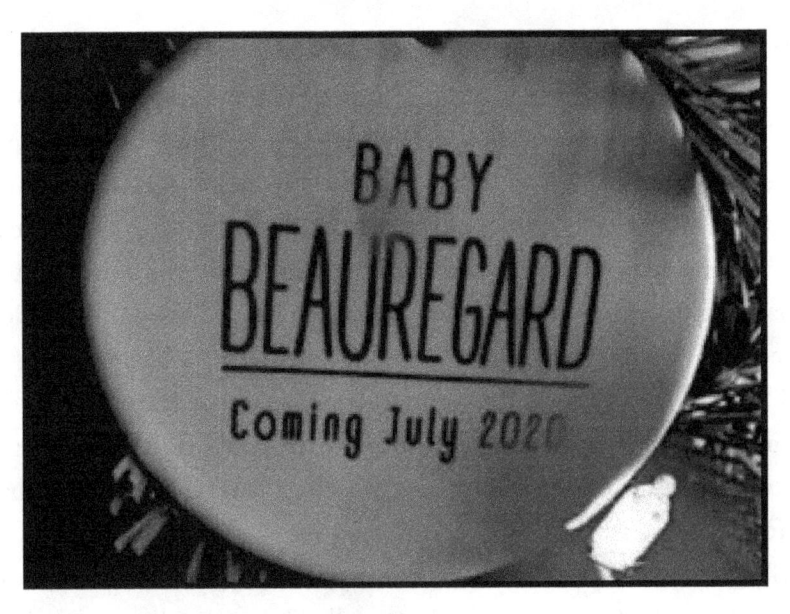

Photo Credit: Kathleen Beauregard

More than 8 million babies in America have been born from IVF since 1978. Statistics show that 55 percent of women younger than 35 become pregnant by IVF on the first try. Amanda later said that when the results came back, the staff at Mass General cheered the good news for her and Patrick. Her due date was July 23, 2020.

During that holiday season, Patrick wasn't on any treatment regimen, and he said he felt better than he had in two years. "Until you're totally off everything, you forget what being NORMAL feels like," he said.

The terrible shadow on our family was lifted again, for a time.

Kathy and I didn't like the thought of Amanda being alone for several days at the hotel and hospital in Bethesda while Patrick went through complex lung surgery and other procedures. He and Amanda were happy to have us accompany them for support. For Kathy and me, it was our second visit to the NIH. We'd been there in 1987 for the NIH trial that my brother and I participated in. We'd even been in the same red brick Building 10, the Clinical Center, where Patrick's procedure would occur.

In a CaringBridge post, Patrick provided a digested version of what was going to happen. "They take out one of the cancerous nodules in my lung. They then tinker with this in their labs for as much time as they need (can be anywhere from 2–8 months) and then call you back down if they find activity in the cells and create a custom treatment for your cancer."

The lung surgery involved a minimally invasive procedure that relied on small incisions between ribs in Patrick's chest. Through one, doctors inserted a slim tube with a fiber-optic camera and a light source at the end. Through two others, they inserted surgical instruments. Guided by the camera, they removed several tumors from his right lung. Through yet another incision, they then inserted a chest tube that would remain in place for several days.

Chest tubes are plastic tubes that are used to drain fluid or air from the space between the lungs and the chest wall. They typically remain in place for two-to-five days or sometimes even longer; removal is often painful. Seventeen years earlier, Dan had endured a chest tube during his junior year at Thayer Academy after developing bacterial pneumonia, which created a lung abscess. He underwent urgent surgery at Mass General and required a chest tube for nearly 10 days. He was not left with any residual breathing problems. Indeed, a few weeks later, he was back on the ice playing highly competitive hockey.

Patrick tolerated the procedure well. "Surgery was a success," he wrote in CaringBridge. "I had two pieces of my right lung removed on Friday and they are confident they got plenty for samples. They actually ended up taking out more than anticipated, and because they went into two different sites it has made the recovery slower. One to two days of a chest tube is turning into four days. The chest tube sucks, but once that finally comes out it will bring much relief."

His tumor samples went to a laboratory for analysis to determine if CAR-T therapy would be a treatment option—they tested to see if the TILs were effective at all against his cancer. Meanwhile, the process of enhancing his TILs got underway. That can take half a year or more. If all goes well, the strengthened cells can be harvested and infused back into the patient. That would require more chemotherapy, given to lower the number of immune cells in the body and then rebuild the immune system from the ground up. That stage of the treatment can take several months.

Facing those prospects, Patrick wrote, "There is also the chance that they find that your tumors show no activity of TILs at all. In that case, to be as blunt as possible, you're basically shit out of luck. This trial isn't for you then. They don't just dump you and leave you out in the cold; they work with you to find something else either there or elsewhere."

As we awaited news about the tumor analysis, I wrote to Kimmie Ng, "We are believing in the hope that's growing in a test tube somewhere in Bethesda."

She responded, "I am also keeping my fingers crossed about the NIH trial. You must be thrilled at the baby news as well—congratulations!"

Though Patrick's recovery from the surgery took longer than expected, by the end of January 2020 he was feeling good and working at his job and exercising again at the gym. While he waited for the NIH results, he was free to participate in another clinical trial, and in February 2020, on the advice of Dr. Ng, he started participating in another at Dana-Farber. The trial combined two novel checkpoint inhibitor drugs considered to be breakthrough drugs for treating advanced malignancies. Though many patients with MSS colorectal cancer like Patrick didn't respond to the regimen, one patient had had striking success.

Of this new trial, Patrick wrote, "This Thursday will be round # 1! The trial consists of 2 different infusions of immunotherapy drugs meant to stimulate my own immune system to recognize and then fight the cancer. The good news is that the vast majority of patients on this trial are reporting little to no side effects. Let's hope that I am in the majority and, even more importantly, the stuff works! I got a good feeling."

On February 7, he was back in the infusion chair at Dana-Farber for a long, tiring day. "We were there from early in the morning until 7:30 p.m.," he wrote. "I had to have vitals taken every 15 minutes throughout the infusions and afterward. I also had to wear a Holter monitor for about 7 hours (it is essentially a mini-EKG machine taking readings of your heart constantly). I also had what felt like my entire body drained of my blood for all the tubes they had to take for research and monitoring."

The next day and over the next week, he had to return for more blood draws. "All of this monitoring is only for the first round or so. The reason is that there is the (low) possibility of these drugs stimulating my immune system and causing it to attack healthy organs (heart, liver, stomach, brain, etc.). This typically manifests itself very early on after the first infusions so it's a good sign that all went well yesterday. Zero side effects as far as I can tell just now."

All of us continued to hope for a breakthrough.

# 15

# The Advocate

WITHIN MONTHS OF Patrick's diagnosis, he had turned himself into a poised and articulate advocate for fighting young-onset colorectal cancer. He joined forces with a range of cancer-fighting organizations, urging earlier detection and raising money for research to improve treatment outcomes. He often made video appearances for the cause. Typically, he would recount his experience. "It was a complete and utter shock to me," he said on a video for the Jimmy Fund, which supports Dana-Farber. "Honestly, I thought I was another healthy 29-year-old." Even after getting the diagnosis, "I was in complete denial," he continued. "There's just no way I'd have this cancer inside me and not know about it."

In all his appearances, he warned his contemporaries to stay vigilant about their health and especially watch for worrisome signs. Awareness was a key—particularly given the lack of obvious early symptoms in many young people with colon cancer. "As far as I could tell, I hadn't exhibited any symptoms," he told a webcast put together by the Cancer Prevention Foundation and the Congressional Families Cancer Prevention Program.

One problem, he acknowledged in the webcast, is that many colon cancer symptoms are generalized—such as stomach pain, cramps and blood in the stool that could be reflexively attributed to hemorrhoids. "I may have exhibited some symptoms before the stomach pain, but I could have just brushed them off, thinking maybe I ate something bad today."

In the spring of 2020, he gave a talk to employees of Boston Biomedical, a biotech company focused on cancer research, during a lunch event at the company's headquarters in Cambridge. "It was a lot of fun," Patrick later told his CaringBridge audience, "and I think plenty of people in the audience were sufficiently scared shitless enough to go get their colonoscopies done."

He also pointed out in the webcast that awareness needs to reach more primary care doctors, many of whom still think of colon cancer as mostly an old person's disease. He told of a friend with symptoms who raised a question with his primary care doctor. The doctor dismissed the concern, saying that the friend was young and in shape, not to worry. "You need to be a strong advocate for yourself," Patrick emphasized.

To help raise funds for research, he worked with organizations from the aforementioned Jimmy Fund (the famous charity founded in 1948 by Dr. Sidney Farber that was named for a Maine boy dubbed "Jimmy" suffering from lymphoma) to the Colon Cancer Alliance to Conquer Cancer, a branch of the American Society of Clinical Oncology (ASCO). He spoke to the Congressional Families Cancer Prevention Program, a bipartisan group of House and Senate spouses that promotes research and awareness. Often joining with Panda Power and Brendan, Patrick participated in or encouraged various fundraising runs and other events. His friends jumped in, too. One friend, who organized annual charity golf tournaments in Falmouth, dedicated the 2018 event to Patrick. The man who trained Patrick's dog, Ruby, organized Paws for Pat, a fundraising dinner in South Boston.

In almost all his appearances, Patrick struck a note of optimism—encouraging others who might be suffering from cancer and expressing hope in his own situation. "If you're still out there fighting like I am, know that you're not alone and keep fighting and never, ever give up," he told participants at the start of one 5K race.

"I'm well aware of the statistics," he said in the Jimmy Fund video. "But there are plenty of people out there who beat stage 4 colon cancer. So, with that, it gives me hope, and I will never give up."

The fight against the growing scourge of colorectal cancer among young adults got a major boost in March 2019 when Dr. Ng helped found the Young-Onset Colorectal Cancer Center in association with Dana-Farber and Brigham and Women's Hospital. One of the first such facilities of its kind in the nation, the center provides affected young adults and their families with a holistic approach to care, including a multidisciplinary evaluation and treatment team, genetic testing, support resources and services. Research is the center's keystone.

Like John E, Kimmie Ng is a member of a special breed of medical oncologists. One of three daughters of parents from Taiwan and Singapore, she grew up in New Jersey. Her initial aspiration was to become a concert pianist and so she studied classical piano for seven years. Ultimately, however, she decided that she didn't want a professional music career to erode the joy of simply playing the piano.

As she became more interested in science, she pivoted to a career in medicine. Although her initial research interest in the molecular mechanisms of malignancy and metastasis led her to laboratory settings, her desire to directly help people grew. After earning an undergraduate degree in molecular biophysics and biochemistry at Yale, she attended the University of Pennsylvania School of Medicine. Then she was accepted into a hematology/oncology fellowship program at the Dana-Farber Cancer Institute. Once there, she sought out a mentorship with Dr. Charles Fuchs, an internationally recognized expert in gastrointestinal cancers and cancer epidemiology.

Medical oncology is stressful. Many patients suffer and die. Dr. Ng knew she couldn't handle the emotional burden associated with seeing individual patients every day. She found relief in the opportunity to help patients on a broader scale on her research days.

Patrick, Amanda, Kathy and I got to meet her husband, Henry Su, a neuroradiologist whom she met on the first day of medical school at UPenn, and their two daughters, Chloe and Siena.

One of the known factors that increases the risk of colon cancer is having a first-degree relative (such as a sibling) with the disease. Accordingly, Dr. Ng recommended that Patrick's brothers and sister undergo colonoscopies—considered the screening test of choice in people at high risk. During 2019 and 2020, each of Patrick's siblings underwent a colonoscopy, and none revealed evidence of any abnormality. Kathy and I exhaled.

In founding the center, Dr. Ng gave regular credit to Patrick. "Patients like Pat are really the underlying inspiration for why we wanted to start a center like the Young-Onset Colorectal Cancer Center," Dr. Ng said.

From the start, Patrick promoted the center and was featured in videos and promotional materials. "Did some filming at Dana earlier today with Dr. Ng," Patrick wrote on CaringBridge in the fall of 2019. "It was a marketing video for the new young-onset CRC center and a video to be played on their Chinese website and will be broadcast in their China market. Dr. Ng spoke some Mandarin while I sat there and pretended to be examined. Look for me on a billboard in Beijing or something." To this day, the center continues to rely on photos of Patrick.

The Boston newspapers and TV stations ran stories on Patrick's advocacy and on Brendan's fundraising effort in the marathon. In the spring of 2020, Patrick drew national attention with an appearance on *The Today Show*, NBC's popular morning program. That event came about through the Colon Cancer Alliance (CCA), a nonprofit that promotes awareness of the disease, support for patients and help with research funding. Patrick worked closely with the group and served on its Never Too Young Taskforce, a committee focused on colon cancer in young adults.

CCA enjoys a close relationship with *The Today Show*, which has been a pioneering advocate for awareness of the disease since Katie Couric, a longtime host of the program, lost her husband to colon cancer in 1998. The show started a campaign to urge screening and runs an annual segment in March on colon cancer. The 2020 program hit particularly close to home because the brother of Craig Melvin, the show's news anchor and co-host of NBC's *Today Third Hour*, had been diagnosed with Stage 4 colon cancer at 39.

Through CCA, Patrick was invited to appear on *The Today Show*. NBC sent a producer and cameraman to South Boston to film a pre-taped portion of the segment, which included an interview of Patrick and Amanda in their apartment and video of them walking in the neighborhood. Then Patrick and Amanda—who was five months pregnant—drove to New York City for a live appearance on set. By then, he had undergone 40 rounds of chemotherapy and was on the clinical trial regimen with Dana-Farber. On March 10, dressed in a blue suit and tie, Patrick looked slender, but healthy, and he spoke with his usual vigor and composure. "I feel great, to be honest with you!" he told Craig Melvin. "I really do. I'm just happy to be here."

With Amanda watching from the sidelines, he urged people to be stronger advocates for their health. When one of the co-hosts, Jill Martin, remarked on the positive attitude that he and Amanda shared, Patrick said, "I don't see the point in being negative in this. Negativity is only going to bring on more negativity. I choose to have a positive outlook and always have hope, and I don't see why you would ever decide not to."

Dr. Ng appeared via a remote feed and restated the grim and mysterious reality of the rise in colon cancer among the young. Of Patrick, she said, "Caring for him has hammered home the urgency of why we need to do this research to understand the risk factors and prevent this from happening in the future. Seeing him turning this into an opportunity and a platform to help other people—there is nothing more selfless and noble."

Watching Patrick appear on national television brought out for me the usual mixture of pride and sorrow. He appeared strong and sounded so articulate and forceful that it was almost possible to ignore his physical decline and forget the circumstances that had brought him all this attention. Almost, but not really.

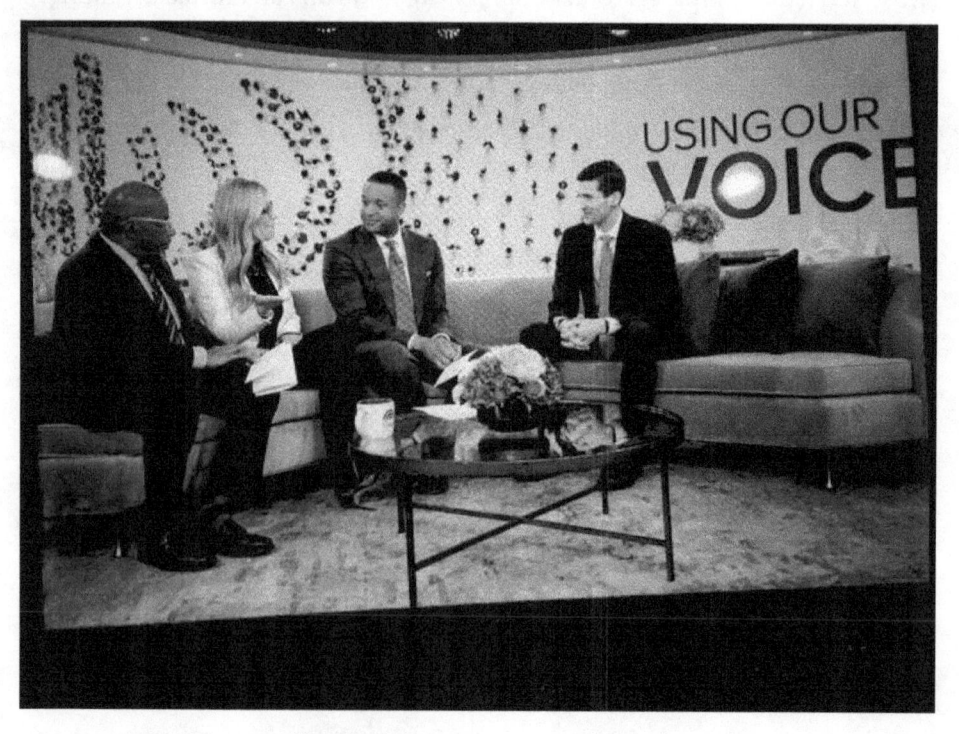

Photo Credit: Nathan Congleton/NBC

Craig Melvin's brother, Lawrence, died from stage 4 colon cancer on Dec. 9, 2020, at the age of 43.

# 16

# Rock Bottom

BY MID-MARCH 2020, the COVID-19 epidemic had descended on the country. Boston ranked among the top five major U.S. cities in the number of cases. The mayor of Boston and the Massachusetts governor ordered schools and non-essential businesses to close. People were urged to socially distance themselves and stay at home. Both the city and state implemented limits on the size of social gatherings. Dana-Farber imposed tight restrictions on visitors entering the facility.

On March 30, after completing the second cycle of the clinical trial, Patrick went alone to Dana-Farber for a full day of laboratory studies and more CT scans. If the scans showed improvement, the next dose of immunotherapy would be administered.

The scan news was bad. The previously existing pulmonary nodules had increased in size and a new lesion had appeared in Patrick's liver. The results deemed him ineligible to continue in the trial. He called Kathy with the grim message, and she put him on speaker phone. His voice was flat. We offered love and support, including suggestions for next steps. Clearly not in the mood for a longer conversation, Patrick told us he was heading back to their apartment. We offered to speak again later in the day if he felt up to it. He said, "Maybe. Love you, too. Goodbye."

Kathy and I stood, initially silent in our shared sorrow and disappointment. Kathy sat briefly and started to cry. I approached her, but she indicated that she wasn't ready to embrace. Once again, rage came over me, but I put the brakes to it. Kathy looked up and declared, "We have to go see him and Amanda. Even if we can't go inside." The lockdown was still in effect.

We drove to their apartment in South Boston. With Interstate 93 North eerily without its usual heavy traffic, we arrived at Patrick and Amanda's apartment on Pacific Street in only 35 minutes, half the time on a normal busy day. Kathy called Patrick's cell phone. No answer. She tried Amanda's phone. No answer. Patrick's car was parked on the street, so he was clearly at home. "They might not be ready to talk just yet," I suggested.

Kathy's cell phone rang. It was Amanda, who appeared in a window of their second-floor apartment, waving and with a somewhat forced smile. She said that Patrick was taking a nap. "We're just here to show our support and love for you two," Kathy said. "We'll always be here." With that, we blew kisses to Amanda and waved goodbye. The ride back to Medfield was mostly in silence.

For the first time in almost a year, Patrick returned to his personal journal. "Do you think when you hit rock bottom, you're able to consciously realize it?" he wrote. "Or is it not until later reflection when we discover it? Because I sure as hell feel like I'm at rock bottom right now.

"Almost a whole year has gone by since I last wrote, perhaps because it has been my most challenging year by far. And it feels like the real challenges are only just beginning.

"Today was the worst news we have heard since the start of this whole thing. The clinical trial lasted even shorter than the last one, this one leading to much more disastrous results. I don't know how many tumors are in my lungs now, I think they gave up counting themselves. They are also much bigger than what they once were—probably why I can't walk up steps and feel winded now. The worst news came in the form of a new discovery of a liver met. This one really shook me because I was not expecting that. I haven't seen growth like this before." In his dispiritedness, he wondered if the lung surgery had fueled the cancer—but that was very unlikely.

"This is the first time I have truly felt like a cancer patient, or that I have cancer," he continued. "I just don't have strength and energy like I used to. I can barely breathe anymore. My ultimate escape was always exercising. It made me feel more alive and reminded me of how capable I still was. That is now gone for me. I still enjoy the challenge, but I am now lightyears away from being capable of what I used to do, even just like 4–6 months ago. Things have not been the same since that lung surgery.

"What hope can be offered during a time like this? Stuck inside our house all day due to coronavirus. How are we to travel to seek out new trials? Are there even any trials accepting right now?

"People always ask you in this situation: 'How are you feeling?' The most honest answer: *Tired.* I'm so damn tired of it all. Tired of thinking about it, tired of having to deal with it, tired of talking about it, tired of it defining my life, tired of being so tired. I feel most bad for Amanda. This isn't the life she deserves, from the one I promised her."

On March 31, 2020, Patrick received a note from the NIH:

"I'm so sorry to hear that your tumors have grown. Hopefully things will clear quickly, so you can enroll in other clinical trials. Please send your scans when you are able. Please also keep us updated with what therapy you and your oncologist decide on. Right now we are essentially closed to treatment as well. However, we are continuing to work on your cells in the lab. We are working on making a T-cell receptor (TCR) therapy for your KRAS 13D mutation. It does not look like we will have a TIL therapy option for you, but we are working on making a T-cell receptor therapy. We are still a while from having anything, but even during this time we are still working on your cells."

Over the next few days, Patrick made several more entries in his personal journal as he clearly tried to buck himself up to continue battling. "I don't have any time to dwell on any of this and sulk or moan for too long," he wrote March 31. "I got laid the fuck out with one of the biggest haymakers I've ever experienced yesterday. But I need to pick myself up off the mat again."

A day later, he wrote, "Time to set a new game plan and push forward. I have felt like absolute shit lately, but I need to keep going and give my body what it needs to improve and heal itself. The last thing I will do is give up. I refuse to die and look back and wonder if I did everything I could to stay here for Amanda and our son. With all this free time on our hands, it's the perfect time to regroup and get motivated to get back into this thing."

The clinical trials had left him frustrated and angry. "But what's the point in dwelling on that now? The past is the past. It's time to move forward. That's all we can do."

But by April 10, his physical deterioration was sinking his resolve. "One of the hardest and darkest days I have had to deal with yet. I just can't even seem to string together a block of good hours let alone a few days. My shortness of breath has become debilitating, and it then affects my mental state. I'm sure some of the breathing issues are in my head and I make it worse on occasion, almost like a panic attack and I feel like I am drowning."

Those were the last entries Patrick made in his private journal.

After Kaylin and Paul got married, in November 2017, Paul's mother gave Kaylin a small wooden prayer box—a container used to hold important prayers and messages of faith, hope and personal intentions. Kaylin used it occasionally. On April 2, 2020, she wrote a sticky note and placed it in the box. It read, "I hope my dad is able to experience some healing while writing his book about our family's battles with cancer."

The following day, she wrote, "I pray that the 9 of us (plus?!) can have a family dinner again soon."

# 17

# "He's Here!"

As spring moved toward summer, the raging COVID-19 epidemic kept most people confined at home and made life especially difficult and awkward for Patrick and Amanda. Patrick was on oral chemo, but still had to go to Dana-Farber for chemotherapy-related tests and procedures. Now he went alone. Amanda was entering the last stages of her pregnancy—they'd decided to name the baby boy Noah—and she had to be particularly careful about avoiding the virus. Kathy and Brendan often shopped for them and after wiping down products with Clorox, dropped off the groceries and other household items, usually on the stairs at the apartment.

Patrick confided to Brendan his concern that hospitals would be so overwhelmed that they'd use triage and bypass late-stage cancer patients such as himself. But he was more outspoken in his aggravation on hearing people complain about the tedium of the lockdown. "Do you want an alternative?" Patrick wrote to his brother. "Okay, then why don't you go volunteer at a hospital and see how bored you may be there. We are sitting safely in our homes while there are so many out there still having to go to work under the anxiety of being outside and in contact with others. There are so many others who are actually sick, others who are currently fighting for their lives inside hospitals. It could always be worse. In the Marines, they tell you to never complain about your current situation. Why? Because right when you bitch and moan, it will get worse!"

In the same message, he quickly reverted to encouragement, presumably meant for himself as much as for Brendan. "It may be difficult, but we must try to keep our minds and bodies sharp during this time. It has admittedly been very difficult even for me. It is far easier to let boredom and laziness take over and just submit yourself to a life of basically nothingness. What is harder is forcing yourself to still get a workout in, still read a book and learn a thing or two and continue to do something (anything!) that is positive and creative.

"Life is different now, but it won't stay that way forever. It is important to remember that this is only temporary, and while it may seem like an eternity now, we will soon be looking back on this time and realizing it was nothing."

Following yet another disappointing update on Patrick's cancer, Brendan responded with his own burst of encouragement. "I cannot imagine what today has been like for you," he wrote. "I cannot imagine what the last 30 months have truly been like for you. Personally, today I felt rage. I felt anger. I felt sadness. The bombardment of thoughts and questions ran through my mind. How? Why? What next?"

Brendan continued, "A man once said: 'Bad news and adversity can wreak havoc on your mind.' But here's the thing. He didn't stop after writing that. He added, 'Yet we have the choice to allow this or not.' I think you are quite familiar [with] who said that. You said it yourself.

"We are in this together. We will always be in this together. No matter what. And I am not doing this without you. You are still here. You still will be here after. Let's get after it."

Despite Patrick's determination to fight on, reality was forcing him to make some hard decisions. In June 2020, he and Amanda decided not to renew the lease on the apartment where they shared so many fond memories. Patrick's declining functional status and uncertain future forced them to make a change. They moved in with Charlie and Roz in Amanda's childhood home in Lowell, Massachusetts. Patrick and Amanda lived on the roomy third floor.

Just over a week later, during a phone conversation with Kathy, Patrick said he wanted to die in the Medfield family home. She assured him that his wish would be honored. No parent should ever have to hear a request like that from a child, but the thought of our son dying anywhere but home was unimaginable.

Brendan recognized how much Patrick was suffering. "By the time of July, everything just seemed off," Brendan later wrote. "Pat was acting differently. He seemed more irritable, not as talkative, and looking thinner and sicker. Amanda, meanwhile, was a couple of weeks away from giving birth. At first, I thought Pat was maybe having heightened stress linked to becoming a father. But then I remember Pat mentioning he'd been having increasing headaches.

"I worried more when I overheard a not-so-pleasant phone call between my dad and Pat. I can recall hearing Pat yell at my father and saying he was fine, that he didn't need to go to the hospital, despite my father's advice. It seemed so unlike Pat."

Patrick had been suffering from chemotherapy-induced colitis, and on June 17, tests showed that the ailment was worsening. Doctors thought that they'd have a better chance to control it in a hospital setting, so they sent him to Brigham and Women's Hospital in Boston. (Dana-Farber Cancer Institute is not an acute-care facility). The Brigham doctors treated him with IV fluids and kept him overnight.

"Thankfully, they recently changed their visitor policy, so I am allowed one visitor (supposed to be the same person) for about 2 hours between 1–8 pm," Patrick wrote in a CaringBridge entry. "I'm sure Amanda is just jumping for joy being almost 8+ months pregnant."

That was the last entry that Patrick made to his CaringBridge journal.

On the evening of July 6, 2020, I was at home when Amanda called. I hoped that she had something to say related to her pregnancy, but her voice projected worry. She told me that over the last hour or so, Patrick had suffered a headache and vomited. I asked if he had a fever, impaired vision, difficulty walking or any other symptoms that would indicate serious trouble. She said they didn't have a thermometer, but Patrick said that he didn't feel feverish. He also had told her that he refused to go anywhere to be evaluated. His tolerance for hospital visits had been worn out. Her answers to my other questions were relatively reassuring. Given that, I asked her to give him some Tylenol and call me back in a couple of hours or sooner if things got worse. But a chyron displaying "brain metastasis" flickered in my mind. I quickly shoved it back into the dark room from where it had emerged.

A couple of hours later, Amanda texted that Patrick was sleeping, and she would get in touch with his Dana-Farber doctors in the morning.

I slowly exhaled.

Early the next morning, Amanda called again, this time sounding very stressed. Patrick's headache had returned, and he essentially hadn't been out of bed for a day due to feeling weak and dizzy. She asked if she should call 911. I said yes. I called her father, Charlie, and asked him if he knew what was going on. He said that Patrick had seemed very tired when they'd chatted the day before. Charlie said he'd go upstairs to check things out.

Later, Charlie told me that Patrick insisted on walking down the three flights of stairs from their bedroom to the house's entryway, where he sat and waited for the EMTs to take him to the nearest community hospital, Lowell General. Soon Amanda texted a dire message. "He's being transferred to Brigham. The CT of the brain apparently showed spots."

A short time later, Kathy and I spoke with Patrick. In a raspy voice, he said, "I just want my son to remember me."

His words weighed like an anchor in the silence.

"Your son will never not know or forget you," I told him. "We, and everyone who loves you and cares about you, will make sure that does not happen…ever. What you need to do right now is put your vision of Noah's face right in front of yours and keep it there. With every ounce of strength you've got, that's what you need to fight for right now. You've been, and will continue to be, a warrior. A Superman. For Noah. For Amanda. For our family. For yourself."

The CT scan of the brain showed multiple metastatic lesions in the cerebellum, cerebral edema (brain swelling) and early evidence of brain tissue, blood and cerebrospinal fluid shifting from their normal position inside the skull. Often fatal if not treated right away, a brainstem herniation is a medical emergency, requiring immediate medical intervention.

At Brigham, Patrick was immediately treated with IV corticosteroids and osmotherapy to reduce the brain swelling. His functional status (such as it was) improved over the next few hours. While the risk of paralysis, coma and death was reduced, Patrick urgently needed surgery to remove the tumors in his brain and provide decompression. Amanda and I spoke on the phone with the neurosurgeon who would be performing the surgery, Dr. Nirvav Patel. Speaking calmly and confidently, he described the procedure with its associated risks and chances for recovery. He never suggested that this surgery could cure the trouble in Patrick's brain.

As much as I wanted to see the scan images, to see if the radiologist's interpretation was somehow inaccurate, I didn't. I knew the odds of inaccuracy were probably close to zero. And I couldn't bear to see those grayscale pixel images turned into living mutations in my son's brain.

That evening, Patrick texted me: "You can't let this break Mom. You have unfortunately seen death throughout your life, she hasn't."

Time stopped. My reaction to those raw, staggering and disheartening words surfaced the same reaction I had when told that Patrick had an apple core lesion. My throat dried and tears streamed down my face. I slowly inhaled, then exhaled, collected myself and responded. "Know that I will do everything in my power to prevent that. As you already know, she is a very strong person."

I decided not to share his pleading text with Kathy or anyone else. Still, I contemplated his remark about seeing death through my life. Although I didn't witness the deaths of my parents and brother, I had seen the before and after of their deaths. I had seen the slow, cruel decline of my brother and father, and my mother's cyanotic, motionless and peaceful appearance shortly after she died. As a physician, I'd seen hundreds of people die or lie at death's door. Some of the deaths were agonizing, others peaceful. Some deaths came quickly—a rapid transition from *in extremis* to the end. Others were cruelly protracted. Some were avoidable, others not.

I knew that death is everywhere, not confined to emergency rooms and intensive-care units, and not just to old people. I had felt the near presence of death in people afflicted with life-threatening illnesses or injuries. I was familiar with the sights, sounds and smells of death. However, the clinical detachment I was trained to have didn't emotionally shield me from my son's suffering.

Later that night, Kaylin prepared an email for Patrick. Very aware that he worried that his son wouldn't know him, she promised him that the whole family would see to it that never happened. To reassure him, she started preparing a list, headed by "Noah will know."

It included:

- that you don't like tomatoes
- that you were unbelievably good at impressions (Grandpa Boris from *Rugrats*)
- that you loved Butterfingers
- that you were the leading example for recruits during your time on Parris Island
- that you admired David Goggins
- that you used to wiggle excitedly while playing video games

- that we were all together in 2017 when the Pats won the Super Bowl
- that you tanned in the summer
- that your nickname was Slug
- that you earned untouchable status as the golden child
- that you could expand your tummy to an incredible size
- that we all loved you incredibly.

Patrick remained at Brigham waiting for the surgery, and on July 9, the hospital made an exception to its COVID visitation policies and let Amanda stay overnight in his room. She had been receiving her obstetrical care at Massachusetts General and her due date wasn't for another two weeks. But during the night, she went into labor. Oncology nurses whisked her from Patrick's room to Brigham's Obstetrical Admitting Unit. Sensing that the baby's arrival was imminent and knowing that Patrick wanted to be present when the baby was born, a nurse decided not to wait for patient-transport services. She put Patrick in a wheelchair and quickly headed to the labor and delivery unit on the third floor of an adjacent building. He missed witnessing the birth of his son by mere minutes.

The news came from Amanda's mother, Roz, via a FaceTime call. "He's here! He's here! Noah has arrived!" she cried.

Momentarily stunned and trying to comprehend what we were hearing, Kathy and I stared at the phone in near disbelief. "What are you saying? Noah's born? Really? Really? Oh, my God!"

Shortly before nine that morning, pictures of Patrick and Amanda holding their newborn son started appearing in text messages and on social media. Patrick looked elated as he cradled Noah, ignoring the port-a-cath clearly visible on the right side of his chest. The scene looked and felt like a miracle.

## GEORGE BEAUREGARD

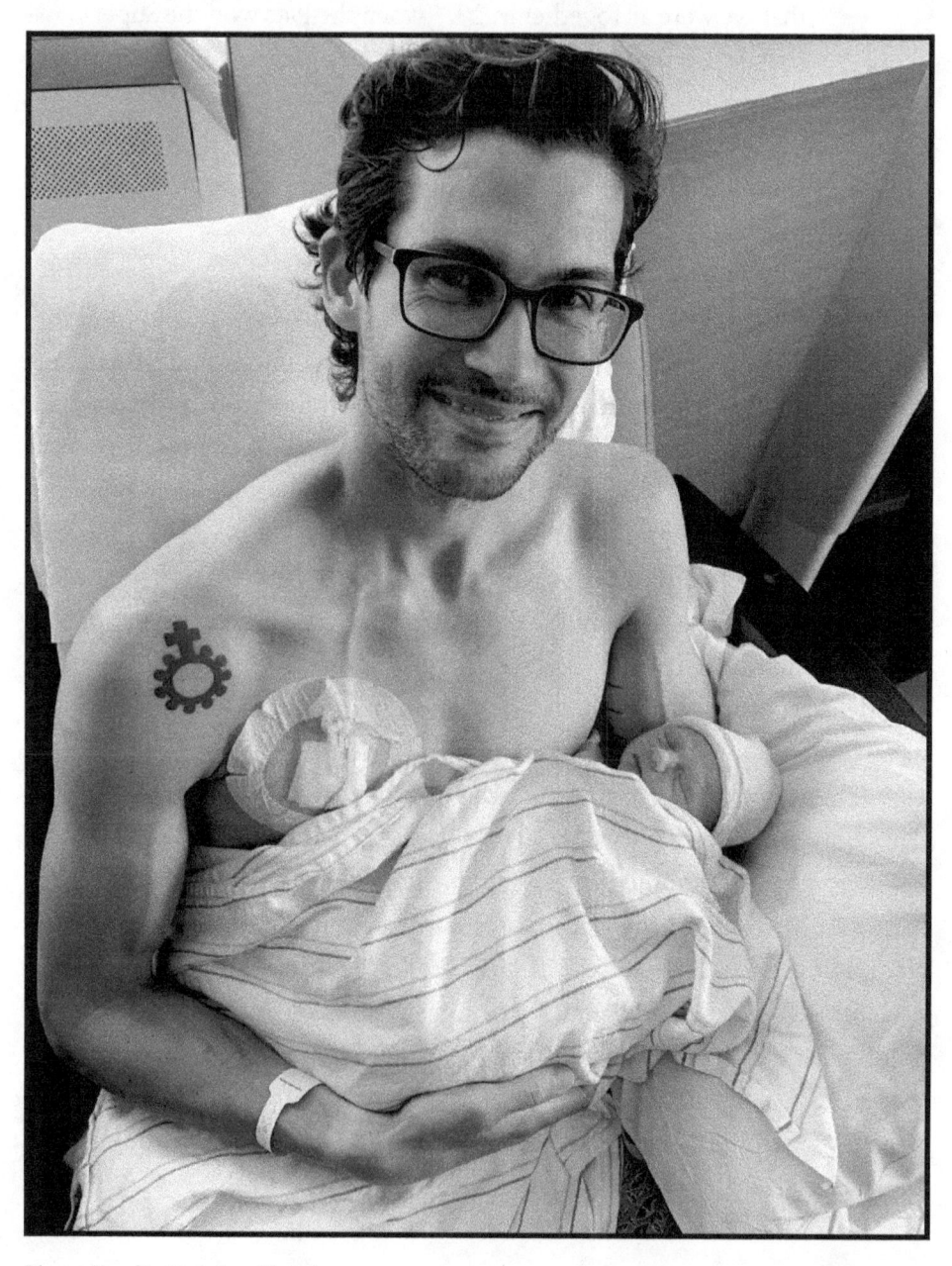

Photo Credit: Rosalyn Flood

Brendan recalled getting the news. "I opened my eyes to see my dad standing at my bedroom door. It was the morning of July 10, and there was a bit of sun shining into the room. "Brendan, someone has arrived," he said.

Amanda had given birth to Noah Patrick Beauregard. When it seemed that darkness was engulfing our family, a ray of light and hope burst in.

To give the new parents extra time to celebrate the joyous addition to their family, a last-minute schedule change moved Patrick's surgery to Sunday from Saturday. Dr. Patel, part of the multidisciplinary team that performed the operation, recalled how the family's story inspired the whole team. "After we decided to postpone the surgery, I explained the situ to the OR team," he said. "To be honest, I wasn't sure how people would react. It was already a busy weekend, and the OR was stretched a little thin due to COVID. But, of course, everyone jumped in to help. The day of surgery, Evan Blaney, the anesthesiologist, turned to me and said, 'Let's do this for this family.' Our patients' bravery makes any challenges we face look like nothing."

On July 12, Patrick underwent a craniotomy and removal of several of the brain lesions, a very delicate and complex surgery. A shunt was placed to drain the extra cerebrospinal fluid that had accumulated. I spent several hours at the Brigham, reading, pacing, and sitting. Finally, I was told that he was out of surgery, which had gone without complications. He was brought back to his neurosurgical intensive care room around three in the afternoon. The head of the bed was slightly elevated, and two layers of thick towels were draped across Patrick's head like a hood. He was asleep, and he looked serene. Over the next hour or two, he would briefly open his eyes, mutter some unintelligible words and then fall back asleep. Eventually, he ascended from the fog of general anesthesia, faced the ceiling and said, "Please stop staring at me. I'm fine."

True to form. Patrick being Patrick.

I smiled and replied, "Okay. I'm here if you need me."

Silence.

Patrick's recovery was quick and without complications. Aside from a sore throat from the endotracheal tube and his frail condition, he felt much better. Becoming a father brightened his temporary recovery.

Behind the scenes, the Brigham care teams, while concurrently navigating the challenges of a high patient census from the COVID-19 pandemic, worked to ensure that Amanda and Noah could stay a few extra days so that the family could go home together.

Later, for an internal Brigham newsletter, Amanda thanked the hospital and particularly the nurses for their kindness. She added that she and Patrick "take each day as a gift—one that has now become even more precious. Any time we get bad news, it's obviously very shocking and so upsetting. But I think we've always tried to stay positive, stay hopeful and keep moving forward. We don't want to fill any day with negativity. We just don't see a point in it, and that's especially true now with Noah. We try to soak up every day together as much as we can."

On July 14, Patrick, Amanda and Noah were discharged. With Noah safely secured in an infant-only car seat, Charlie drove the new family back to the Flood household in Lowell.

Brendan observed that his brother "looked like a new man in so many ways. The first time I saw him, he had shades of relief and rejuvenation. He actually got to be alive for the birth of his son and spend time with him—feeding Noah his bottle and watching TV while the little man napped alongside him."

By now, though, Patrick's physical appearance had changed substantially. He had little hair and had multiple scars on the back of his head. His weight had dropped below 150 pounds. "If Pat was a battery, he seemed to me at 25 percent. And dropping," Brendan wrote.

Next on Patrick's treatment list were sessions of outpatient whole brain radiation therapy. For patients with brain metastases, the treatment is considered palliative, not curative.

Several days before starting the therapy, Patrick asked Kathy, who was visiting him in Lowell, "Mom, can you buzz my head? The back of my scalp is half bald because of the surgery and what's left is going to fall out anyway."

This brought back happy memories of her giving Patrick and Dan crew cuts to start the summer when they were boys. Patrick and Kathy went outside to a second-floor deck. Charlie dragged out a chair for Patrick. Long, slightly curvilinear incisions, the edges closed by sutures and metal staples, tracked up each side of the back of his head. Afterwards, Patrick was pleased. "It looks much better," he told his mom.

When moved to speak about his situation, Patrick could be startlingly candid. Once when Kathy was driving him to a radiotherapy session, he said, "Mom, you can stop doing this. You've got three other kids that need you, too. I'm not going to make it much longer. I'll be okay."

Fighting back tears, Kathy replied, "I'm never going to stop, Patrick. I love all of you the same. Now that you have a son, you'd love any additional children the same. You're my Noah." The exchange continues to haunt Kathy.

Patrick completed the full course of radiation therapy without complications. He soon shared a video of the celebration routine used for patients who had ended this treatment. It showed Patrick standing next to a staff station, wearing shorts, sneakers and a T-shirt with the Marine eagle, globe and anchor symbol across the chest. Masked, he held a short mallet in his left hand. Next to him in a black frame hung a brass Chinese Chau Gong bell. The Chinese believe that the sound of gongs can move people from an alert state (Beta) to a calmer one (Alpha), and ultimately to a meditative state (Delta). On a cue from one of the staff, Patrick struck the center of the gong four times. The sounds were soothing. Staff members cheered and clapped.

# 18

# A Last Cape Vacation

SOMETIME DURING APRIL 2020, Dan and Melissa joyfully told us that they were expecting their first child, anticipated to arrive in mid-October. Another ray of sunshine was heading our way.

We hosted Melissa's baby shower on August 15. We had anticipated that both Amanda and Patrick would be there, but a couple of days before the event, Patrick told Kathy he wouldn't be able to make it. "I'm sorry. I'm just feeling terrible." In the same conversation, he repeated that he wanted to die at home. "Look, Mom, I know I'm not going to survive much longer." He had resumed chemotherapy after the brain surgery, but was between rounds now, and it wasn't clear he would undergo more.

After his brain surgery, Patrick had unexpectedly texted me, "Are you still planning on renting a Chatham house at the end of August?" Given the uncertainty about his condition, I hadn't planned on doing that, but now I embarked on Internet searches for vacation rentals. There was nothing available in Chatham, but a recent cancellation had freed a large oceanfront home in Falmouth, on upper Cape Cod. We would lease the house for the week of August 21–28.

All our children could come for at least part of the week. I knew that this might be Patrick's last Cape Cod vacation, but I was gratified I could fulfill his request.

In mid-August, as our family was preparing to head down to Falmouth, an Amazon package arrived for Brendan. Patrick had sent him a set of noise-canceling headphones. "For a man who was reaching his final weeks, Pat still was looking out for me by making sure I'd be able to focus on doing schoolwork or on a class Zoom call," Brendan later recalled.

Brendan thanked his brother and promised to return the favor.

"No need at all, brother," Patrick replied. "I have no desire for any items, just happy to still be here and spend time with everyone. Excited for next weekend for sure."

We arrived in Falmouth on a Saturday afternoon. That night, Patrick suffered episodic generalized pain that his current medications didn't relieve. I kept some narcotic analgesics hidden in a medication box at home, and so early the next morning, Kathy drove back to Medfield to retrieve some of them; they provided Patrick significant relief.

Overall, the week went well. Patrick ate better than I anticipated, enjoying small portions of snacks, Greek and Italian take-out meals, and wine. Paul cooked a delicious tomahawk rib-eye, which Patrick described as "the best bites of food he'd had in a while." He even managed to spend a day at the beach. During one memorable night, he and Amanda played board games with his siblings and their spouses well into the evening, laughing and telling stories of days gone by.

But the reality of the situation was never far away. On another night, Patrick told Kathy that except for Amanda and Noah being in his life, he would have quit treatment many months before.

Brendan later recalled of the vacation, "The room I was in had an extra bed and one night, I heard my door quietly open to someone slowly getting into it. When I woke up that morning, I saw it was Pat. He mentioned to me he had decided to sleep there since he didn't want to be a burden to Amanda and sit by not being able to help with Noah during the night. I could tell it angered Pat a lot when he was saying that. He would stay in my room for the rest of the vacation.

"Every time Pat went up and down the stairs inside the house seemed like a marathon for him. He would only take some steps before needing to catch his breath and stop for several minutes. The man who had been able to run all the steps around Harvard Stadium with ease and efficiency was now struggling to go up/down a single step. All because of that stupid disease inside killing him."

On one of the final nights in Falmouth, Patrick sent Brendan an email, the last they would exchange. Patrick said his frailty and exhaustion tormented him, particularly his inability to help Amanda with Noah. He dreaded another round of chemotherapy because it made him feel so awful, and he was considering discontinuing it. "Either way," Patrick continued, "I am unfortunately right on the cusp of hospice care and it scares the shit out of me. I have my faith and religion, so I'm not scared to die. I'll be waiting to have a few pops with Pepere and [Uncle] Scotty up there. But I am not ready. I don't want to go. I'm much too young; I'm more afraid of being forgotten. Everyone will be hurt and reminisce on who I was for a couple of years, and then life will go on. People's lives will become busier and busier, and I will just be an afterthought here and there again. It is sad but it is true....

"God chose me, this is my cross to bear. I am not sure why, and going back and wondering why is pointless in my opinion. I am just glad He chose me and not any of you or anyone else in the family. I couldn't bear to see any of you go through this.

"I am very glad we all decided to go down to the Cape; spending time with all of you is a blessing for me. Every day I am still here, while extremely difficult, is a good day. And I intend to stick around here as long as I can."

His condition on our departure day was bad. Looking weak, very thin, unsteady and in pain, he barely made it with assistance to his and Amanda's car. Kathy and I implored him to come home to Medfield. He said he needed to think about when he'd be ready. He'd already decided that the round of chemotherapy he received eight days before the Falmouth vacation would be his last.

His pivot from fighting for life to fighting for time had begun.

Finally, with a heavy heart, I came to accept the reality that in spite of his bravery, tenacity, determination, and optimism, Patrick, like many others with advanced cancer, had faced years of toxic therapies and major surgeries that provided marginal benefit.

That night, while trying to find some bright spots among everything Patrick had endured since his cancer was discovered in 2017, I realized that I had missed a vital one. That slight benefit likely granted him an invaluable extra month or two, enabling him to witness and cherish time with his newborn son.

# 19

# Homecoming

On August 31, Kathy drove to the Floods' home in Lowell to pick up Patrick, Amanda and Noah and take them to Medfield. We decided that they would sleep in our master bedroom on the second floor, which has an attached bathroom. Kathy would sleep in the unoccupied upstairs bedroom. I would sleep on the long sofa in the family room.

The first night was uneventful. Kathy slept with her cell phone by her ear.

Over a couple of days, Patrick's condition deteriorated faster than we had anticipated. Dr. Ng arranged hospice services and ordered items to support Patrick at home. Because the stairs were too much for him, we removed some furniture in the living room to accommodate a large hospital bed. Our first floor has an open plan where the living room and family room are contiguous, with French doors between them.

The living room featured a built-in bookcase with four shelves, each dedicated to one of our children. The shelves held pictures, trophies, figurines, and such. Every item evoked a dear memory.

Patrick's shelf held, among other things, Providence College and USMC mugs, a glass containing some Cape Cod beach stones and shells, a 2016 Northeast Security memorial award, and a picture of him playing lacrosse. Also on the shelf was a small, blue wooden Dala horse that we had bought during a memorable family trip to Stockholm in 2002 to watch Dan play hockey in an international tournament. Dala horses are iconic Swedish gifts and considered a symbol of good luck.

The house needed to accommodate a fair amount of traffic. Roz and Amanda's youngest sister, Devin, joined Amanda (who was on maternity leave) and Noah in the master bedroom. Amanda's father, Charlie, spent a lot of time in our home, but usually left in the evening to drive back to Lowell. Brendan was still living at home and Dan and Kay took time off their jobs and came every day. I was working remotely at the time so, early in the week, I occasionally participated in work-related activities—until shortly needing to clear my entire schedule as Patrick moved toward death. Fortunately, our house has a wrap-around front porch, a haven for anyone seeking some private time or space for a private conversation.

We positioned the hospital bed perpendicular to the large picture window, providing lines of sight to our front yard and the street. But Patrick disliked the appearance of the bed—its reminder of a hospital—and preferred the homier comfort of the big sofa in the family room that accommodated his 6 feet 2 inches. A short table by the sofa held various items—a water bottle, magazines, medications, snacks, Kleenex, etc. Several large absorbent pads were placed under him to handle any accidents.

To keep watch, Dan, Brendan or I would sleep on the hospital bed or the recliner in the family room. Patrick resisted the vigil at first, but then consented. The three of us steeled ourselves for whatever lay ahead. We knew that, if we had been in his condition, Pat would do whatever it took to help us in times of need and/or distress. Dan and Brendan had little to no experience in such medical situations. With my many years of work in emergency rooms and urgent care and inpatient settings, there wasn't much

I hadn't dealt with. But it's obviously very different when it's happening to one of your children.

The Brigham Visiting Nurse Services came regularly and provided hospice care—checking his vital signs, assessing his pain and anxiety, and adjusting his medications for those as needed. They always consulted Amanda, Dr. Ng and me.

The second evening, with Dan occupying the hospital bed, passed without any significant problems, but that didn't continue. One night, Patrick developed an urgent lower-gastrointestinal situation and needed to get from the sofa to the bathroom quickly. Both Dan and I had to keep him upright, as he unsteadily shuffled to the bathroom. Afterwards, Dan put him on his back and carried him back to the sofa.

Patrick's lower gastrointestinal issues persisted, and later, he whispered "I can't help it. I'm sorry, I'm sorry, so sorry," he said. Dan, Brendan and I cleaned Patrick and the sofa. What was most upsetting to me was Patrick's relative lack of reaction to this. Had he been his normal self, he would've been furious and humiliated by such loss of control and the need for help from his father and brothers. In any event, through this and subsequent episodes, Dan and Brendan never hesitated to help.

Patrick had reluctantly agreed to have select friends come by to see him. Given his condition, Amanda felt strongly that the occasion had to be short—certainly not more than two hours total, and not more than two people at a time for only ten minutes per visit.

The event took place on September 3 at our home. The hours were set to start at one in the afternoon and we asked visitors to remain outdoors and wait their turn. Dan, Kaylin and Brendan greeted people as they arrived. When most of the friends had gathered, Kathy and I went outside to talk to them. About 60 people had come.

Facing us were "kids" we'd known for many years. We had followed them as they became adults, graduating from high school and college, getting jobs and marrying. Some had become parents. It was painful to see them under these circumstances, but of course we thanked them for coming and remaining steadfast in their love of and support for Patrick. All expressed varying levels of apprehension, uncertainty and sorrow. Many tried to fight back tears; a few were already crying.

Although almost all of these friends had interacted with Patrick via phone calls, emails, video conferences and social media throughout his ordeal, the pandemic isolation meant that most hadn't seen him for quite some time. Witnessing his condition was traumatic for some. Patrick asked many of them to help look after Amanda and Noah. Not all made it inside, as Patrick, exhausted, called for the visits to stop.

Later on, the thought crossed my mind that, despite the Massachusetts lockdown rules limiting even outdoor gatherings to 25 people, no official appeared at our home with questions about our crowd of visitors.

Patrick's condition worsened that night. I wanted to support him as his father and not as his doctor, but with my knowledge and experience I could administer some of his care. With the support of Patrick and Amanda, I had previously told the visiting nurse that I would provide any medical treatment he needed to keep comfortable. So, periodically I gave him doses of what the palliative-care physician had ordered—predominantly narcotics (for physical-pain relief) and anxiolytics (to relieve agitation and duress).

Around three in the morning, with his level of consciousness declining, Patrick began gasping for air, a condition termed agonal breathing, a sign that death is near. Kathy, Amanda and I gently told him, "Let go Pat. It's okay to let go. Your suffering will be over. There are people there that will greet you. It's okay." Dan, Kaylin, Brendan, Charlie, Roz and Devin were with us in the room. Patrick's labored breathing continued for what seemed to be an hour. Then suddenly, it stopped. His breaths, albeit still shallow, were again rhythmic. His mumbling and the expressions of pain on his face stopped. Amazingly, he now appeared to be comfortably asleep. Seemingly, Patrick had rallied.

But my initial reaction was rage. Looking skyward, I silently asked God why He was allowing Patrick's terminal suffering to continue. "He's been through enough hell. Please take him. Please take him. I'm pleading. Why are you being so cruel?" Everyone in the room during those early morning hours was emotionally drained.

The answer to my questions came later that day.

During the early afternoon, a car pulled up to our semi-circular driveway and a petite woman with a gentle smile, a soft voice and a penetrating gaze entered our house. She called herself Mother Olga and she was wearing a traditional nun's habit. Following introductions, she went to the sofa where Patrick lay semi-awake and a bit incoherent. She knelt on the floor next to him and leaned forward slightly. Kathy gently stirred Patrick awake. Almost instantaneously, Patrick looked alert. He weakly muttered something, and he and Mother Olga briefly talked.

We couldn't hear what they were saying, but Mother Olga's presence exuded serenity and comfort.

As I have mentioned before, I've had mixed feelings about my religion. I grew up in a Catholic household, and we went to Mass every Sunday. I went to a Catholic elementary school, and Kathy and I were married in a Catholic church. Particularly after the Church sex scandals, my actions changed. I only attended Catholic ceremonies when it was necessary, such as for weddings and funerals and the rites of sacraments for my children. Nonetheless, as best I could manage, I guided my thoughts and actions by Christian values.

Patrick didn't share my ambivalence about the Church. He had been a man of great faith from his childhood on. He and Amanda usually attended Sunday services at either Gate of Heaven Church or St. Brigid, both in South Boston. His faith didn't waver after his diagnosis. He read the Bible daily. I admired his courage to maintain—even strengthen—his faith in the face of a terminal disease.

Still, with his suffering, my feelings shifted to anger at God. My doubts and rage—rarely spoken outright—never influenced how Patrick chose to continue pressing forward.

Enter Mother Olga of the Sacred Heart, who had become known for praying with cancer patients and their families. She is the founder and mother servant of a Roman Catholic religious community, the Daughters of Mary of Nazareth. She grew up a Christian in Iraq, where Christians had long been persecuted and where their numbers have dropped significantly during and following the conflicts of the last decades. Nonetheless, she earned strong academic credentials while establishing a record of good works, helping the poor in her war-ravaged country. She earned a Bachelor of Science degree in biology and hematology from the College of Science in Iraq, which has helped her in her work with cancer patients. Later, she earned a master's in philosophy and theology from Babylon College in Iraq, which is affiliated with the Pontifical Urban University in Rome.

She came to the United States in 2001 and received a master's degree in pastoral ministry from Boston College in 2005, the same year she was received in the Roman Catholic Church. For almost a decade, she served with the Catholic Center at Boston University, and eventually the Archdiocese of Boston asked her to create a new religious order. On December 9, 2011, she founded the Daughters of Mary of Nazareth, a community of religious women at the Saint Joseph of Nazareth Convent in Quincy, Massachusetts.

After learning of Patrick's battle from a friend of the Flood family, she connected with him and Amanda. They exchanged text messages from time to time, but Patrick's volatile condition and pandemic restrictions prevented in-person meetings until her Medfield visit.

Mother Olga was deeply moved by Patrick's faith and the Saint Padre Pio motto—"Pray, hope and don't worry"—he chose for his treatment journey. "I was struck by his profound sense of who he is and where he was going," She later wrote. "When I spoke about the journey to Heaven, he said to me, 'I'm ready Mother, but not quite yet.'"

She had met many cancer patients who were miserable and angry about having been attacked by this horrible disease, but she didn't see that in Patrick. "He became a voice for the voiceless," she told me, referring to his efforts to raise awareness about colon cancer. "Because Patrick was a man of hope, as he was approaching the end of his battle with cancer, I wanted to do whatever I could to keep the torch of hope alive in his heart and before his eyes all the way to the end. I came into his and your family's life just to be that voice of assurance from Heaven. I pray and hope that voice was what you really needed."

Her fear for Patrick, Amanda and everyone in our families was that we would be so lost in grief that we would not see God in the midst of our suffering. "That's why I believe the Lord gave me the grace" to serve Patrick.

Before meeting Mother Olga, I had mixed feelings about her visit. I admired how her faith had guided her through the darkness of hatred and destruction in her native land, a region known for decades of violent religious conflicts. Still, I felt hypocritical as a lapsed Catholic about to participate in sacrament ceremonies in my home.

Noah, nearly two months old, hadn't been baptized yet because of Patrick's illness. Mother Olga asked Patrick if he wanted to see Noah's baptism and receive last rites. "Though he was very weak, a strong voice came out of his heart with an immediate response that said, '*Yes!*'" she later wrote. She told him that she would "bring the church" to him.

Because she wasn't sure how much time Patrick had left, Mother Olga offered to have Noah baptized in our family room. She could arrange it for that night.

She left the house and after a few hours returned, accompanied by a young priest, Father Michael Zimmerman, who would baptize Noah and administer several sacraments to Patrick. "One doesn't say no to Mother Olga, nor to a call for the sacraments when they are requested," Father Michael told us.

Standing 6 feet and 7 inches tall, he towered over Mother Olga. They had known each other since his senior year at Xaverian Brothers High School in Westwood, Massachusetts. After graduating from Boston University in 2011, and completing five years of theology studies at the North American College in Rome, he was serving as a parochial vicar of two parishes just outside of Boston.

With all the canonical permissions having been granted, Father Michael baptized Noah and then gave Patrick the Anointing of the Sick, the Last Rites and the Eucharist—all within an hour. And, so, on that day, Noah was born into the Church and Patrick was born into Heaven.

Before Mother Olga left, she told Patrick that while he would never play sports with Noah, watch any of his games, take him to his first day of school, be there for his First Communion, and so on, he was passing onto his son the greatest gift that any faithful father could give to his son: the torch of faith through baptism.

She also did something special for Patrick. Knowing that he would not be there to watch Noah grow up, she started a foundation in Noah's name to help pay for his education. Patrick saw all the documents setting it up and the donations that were already going into that account.

As I reflected about that day, I realized that my long-held negative, or at least very skeptical, views about religious faith—shaped by priest sex-abuse and years of seeing bad things happen to good people—had shifted to the possibility of my believing in a benevolent God and an afterlife again. Only time would tell.

Although I had admired Patrick's resolve, I hadn't deeply understood how my son chose to continue living his faith despite his dire situation. Even though I repeatedly heard him say how grateful he was for still being alive, I hadn't *listened*. While I didn't know how I was going to recalibrate my feelings about my faith going forward, I knew that anger would eventually consume me if I continued with it. I and others would be worse off for it.

Later that night, while watching Patrick's peaceful slumber, I understood why he rallied...and thanked God.

RESERVATIONS FOR NINE

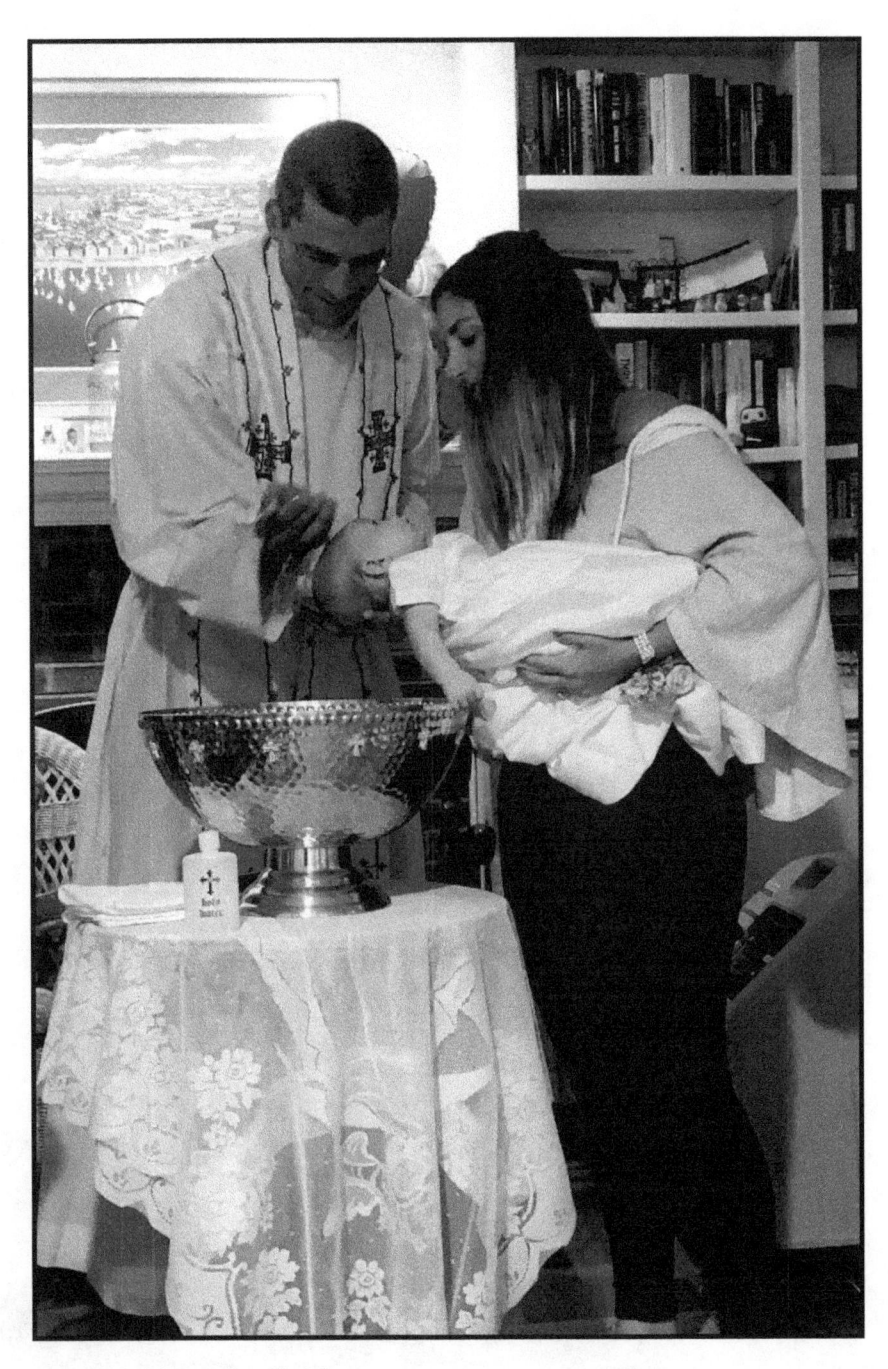

Photo Credit: Rosalyn Flood

# 20

# Taps

ON THE DAY after Mother Olga's visit, a sunny Sunday, September 6, 2020, our dog Mazzy, whom Patrick had trained as a puppy, lay outside on the deck in a lion pose, angled so she could see us gathered around Patrick stretched out on the sofa. She didn't move or bark and looked very, very sad.

Patrick's wife and son, his parents, his siblings, his in-laws and two aunts were present when his battle with early-onset colorectal cancer ended at 12:54 in the afternoon. After his final breath, Kathy closed his eyes, tenderly kissed his forehead, and moved into the foyer, suppressing a deep, raw, agonizing scream—the kind that only a grieving mother could release.

Although there's some relief from knowing that long suffering has ended, words can't describe the grief from seeing one of your children dying in front of you. And before you.

A few hours later, Mother Olga returned. She sat on the floor near Patrick's lifeless body, grasping firmly his limp and cold right hand. She asked that everyone gather near her and began by saying that what we had seen was part of the transition from birth to death, with all the uncertainties along the way. Both involve labor. Patrick was now heading to a better place, one without suffering. It was important that we had let Patrick leave. For those of us who remained behind, our journey would feel like an ocean voyage—sometimes peaceful, sometimes stormy. She finished by saying that it was appropriate for us to feel sad and angry.

Later, someone from the funeral home arrived and removed Patrick's body. A van transported him to Chatham, where Amanda chose to have him buried.

About that day, Dan wrote, "My brother died on our family's couch. I helped the professionals guide his wrapped body from our living room out through the front door and into a van. I thought they might mishandle him—but they never did. They didn't need me. But I still held on to that gurney and body bag—somehow thinking I was helping. Then he was gone."

Over the weeks that followed, no member of our family used that sofa—not even Mazzy. I would occasionally sit in the room and stare at it, sometimes with happy memories of Patrick, other times far grimmer ones. Weeks later, I had mixed emotions when Dan and Brendan removed the couch, cut it into pieces and deposited them into a dumpster.

Because Patrick's final decline had occurred faster than anticipated, many gloomy tasks had not yet been accomplished. Amanda wanted to have him buried in Chatham, where our family had enjoyed many memorable summer vacations and where he and Amanda were married. Amanda had to select a cemetery and plot, choose a casket, arrange times for the wake and funeral Mass, and so on. Kathy and I provided support where appropriate. Chatham is around 100 miles from Lowell and Medfield, so we needed to find a house to rent in Chatham that would be large enough to accommodate both the Beauregards and the Floods. Fortunately, we found one off Main Street. We brought copious amounts of food and beverages and took comfort from the fact that we were all together.

A heavy rain fell during the wake at the Nickerson Funeral Home, in Chatham on September 10. More than 100 people attended, though the mask mandate often made it difficult to recognize who was who. A large-screen television displayed rotating photos of moments of Patrick's life, with large picture boards showing additional memories. Given the crowd, and despite the establishment's best efforts, social-distancing guidelines gave way. People embraced; tears flowed.

Several of Patrick's Marine colleagues attended, some in Dress Blues. Each saluted Patrick's coffin. Dr. Ng came with her husband, Dr. Henry Su, and their daughters, Chloe and Siena. Two nurses, Nina and Taylor, who had cared for Patrick at Dana-Farber also attended.

Inside Patrick's coffin, we'd placed cherished items, such as a piece of the blanket that he carried around as a toddler, one of his baby pictures, a bird's nest, and some small stones that a pair of cardinals—whose monogamous and non-migratory behavior was meaningful to one of his great grandmothers—had mysteriously and repeatedly put on the hood of our car while it was parked at the vacation house in Chatham a year before.

The Mass the next day was held at Holy Redeemer Church, in Chatham. Father Michael presided. Kaylin and Amanda's sisters, Regan and Devin, gave readings. Amanda courageously gave the eulogy, which she had carefully written and rewritten the night before. Throughout, she maintained her composure, as she spoke with elegance and candor.

"Pat fought his disease in the same way he lived his life—with fortitude, grace, and faith," she said in part.

"Reflecting on his life in his final days, Pat said to me that while he wasn't afraid to die, he was troubled and upset because he had always had a feeling that he was destined for greatness. What I told him then and what I share with you now is that he was indeed destined for greatness and that he achieved that greatness by being an advocate and a father.

"So I asked him then and I ask you all now: What could be greater than offering your life to save the lives of others? I believe the answer is being a father. The only achievement greater than saving lives is creating a life. Pat fought hard to be a father. When cancer tried to take him before

Noah was born, he fought back. Emergency brain surgery, intense radiation therapy, and a strong will to live. And that fight allowed him to meet our son Noah and to spend two amazing months with him. The time may have been short, but it was filled with enough love and joy to last a lifetime. I know in my heart that Pat will continue to watch over Noah for the rest of his life and Noah will feel his father's presence every day.

"I ask you to honor Pat's life by reflecting on your own.

Amanda then recited parts of a poem called "The Dash," by Linda Ellis.

The poem reflects on the significance of the dash symbol between the birth and death dates on a gravestone. The poem emphasizes that this small dash represents the entirety of a person's life, encompassing their experiences, relationships, and the impact they made on others.

Amanda concluded by saying, "Cancer took most of Pat's body, but it never touched his loving soul and kind spirit. So, as we say our goodbyes for now to Pat, I ask that you live your dash as he lived his—full of love. His abundance of strength and love will live on forever. We have the best angel watching over us."

At times during the Mass, only my heart, massively weighed down by sadness, prevented me from experiencing another dissociative state or a spiritual plane.

Amanda had chosen Union Cemetery as the most appropriate place for Patrick's burial. A town rule, however, held that only Chatham residents were eligible. Fortunately, a Flood family friend, a Chatham resident, attested that Patrick was an extended family member, which satisfied the requirement. Amanda selected a plot near a flagpole bearing the American flag.

The funeral procession and the burial were steeped in Marine honors. In one sense, it was fitting that Patrick was laid to rest on September 11, recalling the events that inspired him to become a Marine. The hearse carrying Patrick's body featured the USMC eagle, globe and anchor emblem and insignia. At the Chatham Fire Department station, a ladder truck parked outside displayed a large American flag and firefighters stood in formation

# RESERVATIONS FOR NINE

and saluted the procession as it went by. Chatham Police Department vehicles were stationed at intervals along the route with their lights flashing. Police officers stood at attention and saluted the procession.

Instead of taking the direct route to the cemetery, the procession—in a detour close to my family's heart—drove by the Chatham Bars Inn, where we had spent so many happy and memorable hours in summers past.

Three uniformed Marines awaited us at the gravesite. Taps pierced the quiet. One of the Marines walked to Amanda in her chair while holding a folded American flag across his chest. "On behalf of the President of the United States, the United States Marine Corps, and a grateful Nation, please accept this flag as a symbol of our appreciation to your loved one's honorable and faithful service," he pronounced.

While pride filled my heart, another emotion that I couldn't express did as well. There are words that describe someone who has lost a spouse or a parent. There isn't one for someone who has lost a child. It's that bad.

As I watched Patrick's coffin descend slowly into the grave, my broken heart followed.

Mother Olga had told me once that Patrick's journey was God's plan for him since he was conceived. I had great difficulty accepting that statement. I later asked her to explain what she meant. "I didn't mean that this was God's plan for Patrick to get colon cancer at such a young age and die from it only two months after his first child was born," she told me. "My statement on God's plan was more related to the way that Patrick passed into Eternal Life. During those last 48 hours as I witnessed Patrick's journey to the threshold of Heaven, it's almost as if I was watching him get closer to the gate of Heaven and how God orchestrated the smallest details to make that evening (of the last rites and baptism) happen for Patrick and Noah. I knew only God can make such a thing happen. That is what I meant by God's plan for Patrick, to see his baby boy baptized right before his eyes and for him to receive the Holy Communion on the day of his son's baptism.

There were so many moments in that evening that were extraordinary beyond any human planning."

She added: "Often, in such intense times of grief and suffering, people ask me, 'Why did God allow such a thing to happen?' And I often say that the better question to ask is, 'Where is God now?' It is true that we do not understand why bad things happen in life, even for good people. But one thing I am sure of is that we are never alone. As his biological father, you wept when you lost Patrick, and our God as his Heavenly Father embraced Patrick at the gate of Heaven so that his soul, his body will rest in peace after such a long journey of pain and suffering."

Mother Olga's response brought me solace and eased my rage at God. Though I've had a conflicted relationship with the Church, at least, since the priest sex scandals, Mother Olga's example helped steer me back toward the compassion and mercy that underlie the faith. As a middle-aged man of science, I don't take the Bible literally and consider notions of heaven and hell more as metaphors. Still, I often find myself imagining that Patrick is looking down on me, checking in, urging me on.

Following Patrick's death, tributes from Boston news outlets, national cancer foundations, professional medical organizations and others quickly appeared. The U.S. House of Representatives provided a heartfelt testimonial as well.

Mark Ockerbloom, an anchor at Boston 25 News, who had lost a brother at 46 to colorectal cancer, said of Patrick: "His legacy will be of courage, grace and positivity." A statement from The American Society of Clinical Oncology read in part: [Patrick] dedicated the last three years of his life to raising awareness of colorectal cancer in young adults, a cancer he admitted to not knowing anything about prior to his diagnosis."

On September 15, in parts of a speech delivered to the House of Representatives, Massachusetts Congressman James P. McGovern said, "[W]e ought to live our lives as 'Men and Women for others.'...Patrick embodied this idea in every way.... [H]e saw an opportunity to do good. He used his voice to speak out and bring the issue of colorectal cancer to the attention of researchers, donors, elected officials, and other young people at risk for this disease.... [H]e was a very good man who did his best to serve those around him and made our world a better place."

It's well known that people don't remember most of their dreams. Nonetheless, I've occasionally wondered why I don't remember dreams about Patrick as often as I thought I would. Of the few I do recall, a vivid one stands out. During the early morning hours, wearing his Marine dress blue uniform, Patrick walks into our bedroom, looks at me, and says, "I'm fine Dad. I'll see you again." Before I can respond, he turns and leaves the room.

I was shaken at first, but now I think of that dream a lot.

## 21

# Giving

JUST OVER A week after the funeral, our family visited Mother Olga at the Saint Joseph of Nazareth Convent near downtown Quincy. As we pulled into the parking lot, Mother Olga greeted us with a wave. She gave us a tour of the modestly furnished building and introduced us to several of the other Sisters—eight live there, including Mother Olga.

Then she gathered us in a large room and told us that she had something for each of Patrick's immediate family members. For me, she had a picture of Patrick, taken just before his marriage. He was dressed in his wedding suit with the harbor in the background. His eyes shone and he was flashing a joyful smile. Mother Olga had placed the photo in a tabletop frame. Next to it was a painting of a white flower and the words: *"Those we love don't go away, they walk beside us every day, Unseen, unheard, but always near, still loved, still missed and forever dear."*

To Kathy, Mother Olga gave a silver necklace from which dangled a heart decorated with an amethyst-colored jewel (Patrick's February birthstone) and the words: *"I'll Hold You In My Heart."*

Each of Patrick's siblings received a stone plaque with yellow stars and Patrick's name. Below the stars were words reflecting each of the siblings' feelings about Patrick, as told to Mother Olga.

I was overcome by a mix of sorrow and joy. As only she could, Mother Olga had remembered what each one of us had said to her several weeks ago about how we wanted to remember Patrick.

The picture of Pat still sits atop the table whenever and wherever we have a family dinner.

We returned to the convent a month later for a commemoration of the 40th day after death. The ceremony has a long history in Catholic doctrine and marks the day when the deceased enters heaven, but for us it was an occasion to grieve together and remember Patrick. On that 40th day, Father Michael and Mother Olga led a memorial service and the sisters served a delicious meal.

Like Mother Olga, Father Michael has maintained a special connection to our family. "I've felt close and even a part of the Beauregard family," he told me at one point. "Everyone comments on similarities between Patrick and myself, including our height. Anointing and burying Patrick was also very personal to me because we are the same age and have very similar upbringings."

Since then, Father Michael has presided over baptisms, memorial Masses and catechesis dinners with Patrick's siblings, their spouses and Amanda. In 2023, he presided over the wedding of Amanda's youngest sister, Devin.

Friends of Devin made their own contribution to the memory of Patrick. They arranged to plant a Kwanzan cherry tree on the grounds of Chatham Bars Inn, where Patrick and Amanda celebrated their wedding reception. We call it Patrick's tree. It faces the east, just to the right of the Inn's front entrance.

Kathy and I knew that Patrick would want us to continue our tradition of hosting Christmas Day for our immediate and extended family. Charlie and Roz Flood accepted our invitation to join us for Christmas 2020. After settling in, Roz gave Kathy a large bag in which were several small, wrapped gifts.

Within each was a small bright blue box on whose cover was the pentagon-shaped Superman symbol and inside a pair of Superman Shield cufflinks and a note from Michael Flood, the youngest of Charlie's five siblings.

"In his darkest time a man—a superman–showed us how to live," the note said in part. "He taught me to make every adversity an opportunity. He showed me to link the good and the bad in life. He taught me to understand the tapestry of our lives, to embrace our experiences. To be proud and kind. To be a point of light that safeguards others."

Since Patrick's death, several people and organizations have continued his campaign of education and resources to fight colorectal cancer. On May 5, 2021, Amanda established the Patrick Beauregard Foundation. Based in Lowell, the foundation is dedicated to defeating early-onset colorectal cancer through education, advocacy and collaboration. In particular, the foundation supports the work of Dr. Ng and the Young-Onset Colorectal Cancer Center at the Dana-Farber Cancer Institute.

Joy Saunders, a marketing person for Kendra Scott, a large-luxury jewelry company, came across the Patrick Beauregard Foundation while searching for nonprofit organizations to partner with the company. Saunders reached out to Amanda and the partnership began during Mother's Day weekend in 2021 with a fundraising event at the Kendra Scott store in Dedham, Massachusetts. Twenty percent of every purchase benefited the foundation. Among all the jewelry and items offered was the Panda Power Signature Collection, in which pieces of the jewelry could be custom engraved with words like "Pray, Hope, Don't Worry" or "Panda Power". Two additional events have been held since then—another at the Dedham store and one on Newbury Street in Boston.

To date, the foundation has raised hundreds of thousands of dollars.

Team Panda has also stayed active. Five times it has participated in the Pan-Mass Challenge, a Massachusetts bike-a-thon from Sturbridge to Provincetown, which raises money for Dana-Farber and is recognized as the world's single most successful athletic fundraiser. In 2023, the team wore

Patrick Beauregard Foundation jerseys. Some riders had stuffed pandas fixed atop their bike helmets.

Brendan graduated from Emerson in December 2021, and six months later he became the marketing and communications coordinator at the Joe Andruzzi Foundation, based in North Attleboro, Massachusetts. Andruzzi is a former National Football League player whose career ended after he was diagnosed with a rare and highly aggressive blood cancer. He established the foundation to help patients of all ages struggling with financial hardships after a cancer diagnosis.

In a fundraising video for the Andruzzi Foundation, Brendan cited his gratitude to those who had helped Patrick and our whole family as they faced cancer. He said that as someone who as a child had watched his dad confront cancer and who as a college student witnessed his brother's cancer fight, he saw how the support of others provided help and hope. Working for the Andruzzi Foundation, he added, was like "paying it forward."

The greatest joy for all of us has been the expansion of our family. Dan and Melissa's first child, Camden Patrick Beauregard was born on October 1, 2020, just weeks after the death of Patrick. Their second child, Isabelle Catherine, arrived on December 22, 2022. Kay and Paul have also become happy parents—Miles Patrick Nimblett was born on August 2, 2021. Father Michael baptized Camden and Miles together.

## 22

# Frontiers of Hope

ON MARCH 4, 2023, Dana-Farber's Young Onset Colorectal Cancer Center held its Fourth Annual Patient and Family Forum at the Hotel Commonwealth in Boston. The forum, a series of free educational events for patients and their supporters, featured a variety of speakers, including patients, caregivers, researchers and other medical experts. Patrick's picture was on the cover of the event's brochure.

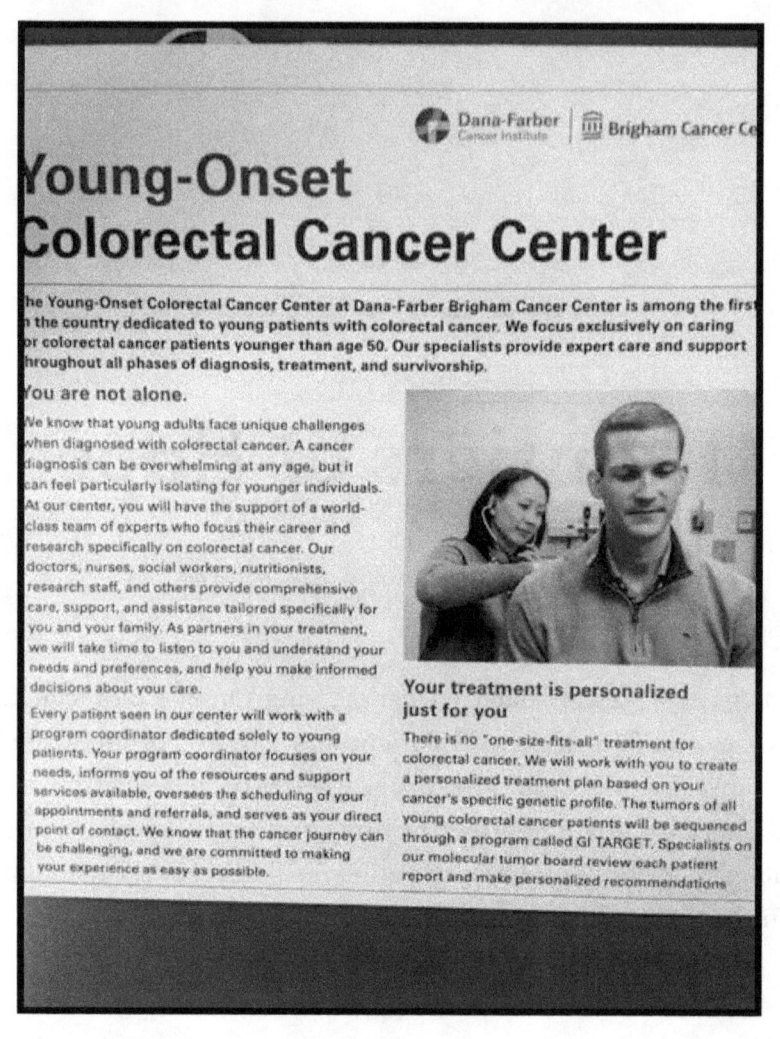

Dana-Farber Cancer Institute, July, 2022

I anticipated that attending would be emotionally difficult, but I knew I had to go and quickly registered. Kathy initially felt the same way, but she also ultimately registered. Though the event was live-streamed, we attended in person. Two women from New Hampshire in their thirties joined us at our table. One had just completed a round of treatment for stage 4 of the disease; the other was her spouse/caregiver. They had a four-year-old son. When a slide from the Patrick Beauregard Foundation flashed on the large screen, they asked if we had a connection. Their expressions turned solemn when we explained who we were.

Since its launch, in 2019, the center has treated more than 700 young patients. While most of these patients live on the East Coast, an increasing number now are coming from around the country. The stories told by patients and caregivers were raw and emotionally draining. But many were also inspiring. These were tales of young adults facing extraordinary physical and mental duress with fierce tenacity.

In any case, I've come to believe that sharing grief provides comfort.

The experts offered updates on new therapies, and some of them show considerable promise. Dr. Myriam Chalabi, an expert associated with the Netherlands Cancer Institute, gave the keynote address for the forum's research section, which primarily focused on advances using checkpoint inhibitors. She described how a neoadjuvant immunotherapy doublet regimen she'd designed had shown strong pathologic responses—with increases in survival rates—in 100 percent of a large cohort of patients with two unique subsets of colorectal cancer.

Several medical experts from Dana-Farber provided news on current research, including clinical-trial findings. Researchers have seen advances in diagnosis and treatment through genetic testing of people and tumors. Other speakers referenced Herceptin, the immunotherapy drug that Jack E, thinking out of the box, recommended for off-label use in my therapy. I wondered if that's what saved my life. Based on what I heard that day and many other studies that I've read, I believe now that environmental factors, such as toxins on the land my childhood home was built on, may have caused the cancers in my adoptive parents and perhaps even me. Of course, germline factors (genetic material passed onto offspring) could have contributed as well.

In her closing remarks for the conference, Dr. Ng reiterated optimism for continued advances in diagnosis and treatment. I left the forum thinking that, had Patrick's cancer come two to three years later, he probably would have benefited from some of the new treatment advances of the past couple of years.

One particularly promising area of research mentioned at the conference concerned the microbiome, the body's ecosystem of microorganisms. These human florae, such as bacteria, viruses and fungi, amount to nearly 40 trillion microorganisms. More than 97 percent of them are in the gastrointestinal tract, especially in the colon. They play an important role in maintaining good health and have been found to mediate a wide range of physiological functions, including immune system development.

Under some circumstances, they also contribute to illness. In the late 1980s and early 1990s, a bacteria known as *Helicobacter pylori (H. Pylori)* came to be recognized as a major risk factor for the development of gastric cancer. (It is also implicated in some stomach ulcers that don't lead to cancers.) *H. Pylori* is detectable via a breath, blood or stool test, and if detected, can be cured by a combination therapy of antibiotics and a stomach-acid-lowering medication.

Currently, the Western-style diet is recognized as a significant contributor to gut microbial susceptibility, chronic inflammation, and various chronic diseases, particularly those impacting the cardiovascular system, overall metabolism, and gastrointestinal health. Abundant evidence links the gut microbiome with colorectal cancer, particularly by affecting the immune response to tumors. For example, research has shown that a bacterium known as *Fusobacterium nucleatum*, which is implicated in causing periodontal disease, is present in colorectal cancer cells and has a causal role in CRC. Conversely, the bacterium known as *Ruminococcus bromii* might improve survival rates.

As Dr. Christoper Lieu, of the University of Colorado Cancer Center, has said, "Alterations of the bacteria and fungi that exist in our guts may lead to an environment where cancer has a higher chance of developing, so physicians and researchers are looking at the factors that may be altering its makeup." A number of factors can be at play in altering the microbiome, including lifestyle changes and environmental exposures over several decades. The mystery deepens because, as Dr. Lieu points out, the increase in CRC has turned up in countries around the world, representing a variety of diets.

Studies have also looked at the microbes inside the tumor microenvironment. It has been demonstrated in mice that these microbes may contribute to the development of cancer, as well as affecting—favorably or detrimentally—the efficacy of various cancer therapies.

These findings could have a profound role in treating colon cancer. Therapeutic resistance and bad side effects currently serve as major obstacles to the effectiveness of certain chemotherapies and immunotherapies. Research indicates that variations in the efficacy of oxaliplatin among patients may be related to biochemicals in gut microbes. What's more, gut microbes have been associated with increasing the toxicity of chemo drugs; modulating the components of those microbes may alleviate the toxicity. It's even possible that pretreatment with targeted immunotherapies might spare CRC patients from having chemotherapy and/or surgery. The same promise holds true for other cancers as well.

Despite a growing body of evidence in human subjects, clinical interventions targeted at the microbiome have yet to be translated from research labs to patients with cancer. Still, the potential exists to modify the composition of the gut microbiome to improve outcomes. And some of the interventions could obviate the need for drugs. Certain changes in eating habits, such as intermittent fasting or high-fiber and keto diets can also alter the gut microbiome.

"The research into what the role of the gut microbiome is in young-onset colorectal cancer is still in its infancy," Dr. Kimmie Ng said recently.

A new study compared both young-onset and later-onset CRC patients to young and healthy people in the control groups. The findings suggest that the patients with cancer had fewer species—and slightly different organisms—in their gut microbiome. Young-onset CRC patients had slightly different organisms than the older-onset cohort.

"This is still just hypothesis generating," Dr. Ng said of the study, "and the results need to be further investigated and validated in larger studies." She went on to say that an international cohort of young-onset CRC patients is being compiled so that researchers can study serial blood and stool samples as they are correlated with clinical and diet/lifestyle data. The effort will allow a robust global investigation "so that we understand how different environmental exposures may be contributing to risk of young-onset CRC," Dr. Ng said.

Another hopeful development: The prevalence of KRAS mutations in CRC patients runs from 30–40 percent. Among the mutations are four major variations. A small percentage of patients have the specific KRAS mutation that afflicted Patrick. As I mentioned in his case, the presence of a KRAS mutation, considered "undruggable" due to its structure, is linked to treatment resistance and worsened survival rates.

But evidence has revealed that not all KRAS mutations are created equal—they vary in responsiveness to different drugs. Recently published clinical trials have demonstrated that therapies targeted at certain KRAS mutations—including the type that Patrick had—can inhibit cancer growth. In addition, the recent discovery of a novel pan-KRAS treatment provides hope for any patients whose cancer exhibits a hotspot KRAS mutation.

Most cancers are detected at later stages, when response to treatment lessens considerably. Dr. Azra Raza, a leading oncologist, researcher, and author of *The First Cell: And The Human Costs Of Pursuing The Last*, has repeatedly said that "People don't die from cancer. they die from late treatment".

In 1962, the famed pediatric pathologist Dr. Sydney Farber expressed a desire for a method for cancer detection before the development of signs and symptoms.

In terms of diagnosis, new developments for detecting various kinds of cancers earlier may have a particularly promising application for colon and rectal cancer, which frequently develops with few if any obvious symptoms. Over the past few years, scientists from several companies have created novel genomic tests for detecting DNA-fragment modifications, genomic alterations, aberrant methylation and certain biomarkers circulating in the bloodstream from cancer cells and tumors—the so-called multi-cancer early detection (MCED) test. Also referred to as a liquid biopsy, it can screen for more than 50 types of cancers. Several large, prospective observational cohort studies have shown promising results in the reliable identification of cancer, often at an earlier stage, when the potential for curative treatment and thus fewer deaths is greater.

Overall, across 50-plus cancer types, one study demonstrated that, in people who had a cancer signal detected, The specificity (true negative rate) of the MCED test was slightly above 98 percent, while the sensitivity (true positive rate) was about 66 percent. The positive predictive value—its precision—was 43 percent. In people who had a cancer signal detected, one study found that the test had more than 80 percent sensitivity for colorectal cancer, while giving few false positives. That notwithstanding, sensitivity increased with stage, meaning that the rates were significantly less in people with lower stage disease.

So far, some medical authorities have seen the viability of an MCED test as a promising complement to, but not a replacement for, colonoscopies and stool tests. Although the initial findings suggest a potential breakthrough in the test's ability to detect cancers at an earlier stage, research is underway by investigators across the National Cancer Institute and at other federal and international agencies to determine their fidelity and clinical utility. Potential pitfalls include false positives that could lead to overdiagnosis that results in unnecessary and invasive procedures. Those unintended consequences are counter to the Hippocratic principle of "first, do no harm".

Conversely, false negatives might result in individuals having exaggerated optimism about their health status and choosing not to follow current evidence-based effective screening recommendations.

Accordingly, some researchers argue that large randomized controlled trials should be conducted to assess whether multi-cancer early detection tests reduce mortality—cancer-related and/or all-cause—before FDA approval and clinical use, to ensure a favorable risk benefit ratio. While I understand their viewpoint, such studies would take years to produce reliable results.

But the undeniable, current reality is that early-onset cancer rates continue to rise, leading to significant suffering and potentially avoidable deaths. So sticking strictly to scientific-research orthodoxies that have been in place for many decades isn't the best approach. Some of my fellow physicians and I believe that erring on the side of over testing is a perhaps warranted approach under this circumstance.

Moreover, is overall mortality the best measure of success? Detecting cancers at early stages, where treatment can greatly improve both longevity and quality of life, clearly offers benefits. Perhaps demonstrating a shift towards detecting more early-stage cancers (the so-called "stage shift") would be a better endpoint. Regardless, whether these tests will revolutionize cancer screening and care remains to be seen.

That notwithstanding, the implications for how this approach to cancer screening, when approved, will affect people and physicians—primary care doctors and oncologists alike—will be profound.

Meanwhile, treatments for the disease that altered my life—advanced bladder cancer—are advancing at a good clip. When I was diagnosed in 2005, the first-line treatment recommendation was radical cystectomy—removing and replacing the bladder—along with chemotherapy. Back then, the five-year survival rate for advanced stage was about 50 percent—and it hasn't improved much since then.

But several studies have recently demonstrated encouraging results using immune checkpoint inhibitors in addition to chemotherapy administered before removal of the bladder. Patients who responded well to the regimen could continue without cystectomy. At 30 months of follow-up, the patients who elected against cystectomy were found to have longer metastasis-free intervals and improved survival rates.

People who've had their bladder removed know how life-changing the procedure is. Our lives would be considerably different if we'd had a proven bladder-sparing option available.

Lately, there's been more good news for sufferers of bladder cancer. A recent Phase 3 study showed that a new combination of treatments—engineered tumor-targeting antibodies and chemotherapy drugs called antibody-drug conjugates (ADCs)—reduced the risk of death by more than 50 percent. Other trials involving the use of ADCs in breast cancer show promise as well. Of the findings related to the use of these weaponized antibodies, a researcher said, "It's going to launch a thousand ships."

Although many additional studies are needed, the preliminary results of these assorted areas of research give me hope for life-saving advances in diagnosing and treating these devastating diseases.

On another front, however, I'm concerned about a recent controversy. In the last few years, both the American Cancer Society and the U.S. Preventive Services Task Force, which consists of volunteer healthcare experts, recommended lowering the suggested age for starting colorectal cancer screening to 45 from 50. The screening could be accomplished by any of the currently available methods—including a stool test done at home—and tailored to the patient's clinical situation.

But in August 2023, the American College of Physicians (ACP), the world's largest medical-specialty society, disagreed, advising against CRC screening in asymptomatic average-risk people younger than 50. In an additional statement, the ACP referenced the low numbers of new cases detected with the lowered age (35 per 100,000) and translated that into gaining five to six additional life days per person screened. Those numbers were described as providing an "inadequate net benefit to warrant screening in average-risk adults aged 45 to 49 years."

Despite statistics indicating a 45 percent rise in young-onset colorectal cancer over the last 15 years, the ACP believes that the risk is exaggerated, with a leading ACP member claiming the reported risk is overstated.

The ACP argues that not lowering the recommended age may lead to a more objective and fact-based evaluation of the risk/benefit ratio of CRC screening. The organization is apparently concerned about harm from colonoscopies as well as about financial costs. Given the low incidence of CRC in young people, the ACP statement argued that a large number of them would need to be screened to prevent a single case of colorectal cancer.

In addition to the advice against lowering the age to begin screening, the ACP also weighed on the value of the two kinds of home colon cancer tests. One, the so-called FIT test, looks for blood in the stool. The other, the DNA stool test, looks for worrisome DNA. That test is more expensive. The ACP advised against use of DNA stool testing as a screening method, citing lack of evidence that it is appreciably more effective.

The Colon Cancer Alliance immediately objected to the ACP recommendations. "Colorectal cancer screening through colonoscopy is a routine and safe procedure," the CCA in its rebuttal said: "Studies estimate the overall risk of complications for routine colonoscopy to be low, about 1.6%." (Complications include bleeding, infection or perforation). "The Alliance advocates for all evidence-based, validated screening methods, including stool-DNA tests. Among their various benefits, stool-DNA tests can improve screening access in underserved communities."

Michael Sapienza, CEO of the Colorectal Cancer Alliance, added, "ACP's actions are regressive and put lives at unnecessary risk. We're finally breaking through the stigma that has long been associated with colorectal cancer, and we're finally addressing its impact on younger people. Now is not the time to make conflicting recommendations or [to] exaggerate the risk of screening. The greatest risk people face today is not getting checked for colorectal cancer."

Despite the controversy about expanding the screening age, Dr. Ng's unrelenting focus remains on "the urgency of the research to figure out what the causes of young-onset CRC are so that we can identify young patients who are at high risk and target them for earlier screening."

I entirely agree with the CCA. Although it's been well established that screening for colorectal cancer saves lives, the actual rates fall well short of the nationally stated goal of 80 percent of the eligible population.

Among other things, prevention is only one goal related to testing for this disease; detection of an existing cancer at an earlier stage that might be curable—or prolong quality survival—wasn't mentioned by the American College of Physicians. What's more, because many people are reluctant to undergo a colonoscopy, an alternative, non-invasive form of screening—such as the stool-DNA test—is better than no screening at all. It's often said, "The best screening test is the one that gets done."

During my clinical career, I was able in a calm and dispassionate way to deal with people who had health disasters. Dispassionate is something I can no longer be about this disease.

Today, first and foremost, I think about my son and the 19,550 people that the ACS estimated will be diagnosed with early-onset CRC in 2023 and the 3,750 who will die within five years. The ACPs position seems to ignore the real magnitude of this phenomenon. The increase in young-onset CRC is expected to continue, such that nearly a quarter of all rectal cancers will be diagnosed in people under 50 by 2030. CRC is also predicted to become the number one cause of cancer-related death by 2030 in people 18–49 years of age (in fact, it is already the leading cause of cancer death in young men). While the statistical life-years gained and mortality reductions may seem trivial, it ignores the personal—the thousands of patients and families affected.

So, I urge all average-risk people aged 45 to 49 with or without non-specific gastrointestinal issues (especially the former), to have a conversation with their doctor about the current risk and effectiveness data on CRC screening. It needs to be a shared decision-making process. If a desire to be screened for CRC exists following the discussion, the next step is learning about what screening options are currently available. Strong evidence exists that colonoscopy and fecal immunochemical test (FIT) are the most effective screening methods. I implore physicians to advise screening for every eligible patient—and to not think of colorectal cancer as a disease confined to older adults with a trivial rise in people under age 50 that doesn't warrant evaluation.

Emerging blood-based tests are now an option for individuals who consistently decline colonoscopy or stool test. If the individual is amenable to having the test, there needs to be an understanding and acceptance that an abnormal test result will necessitate a follow-up colonoscopy.

One final note about medical breakthroughs. Fifteen or so years ago, while researchers were mapping the human genome, many scientists thought the path to victory over cancer would come by targeting specific mutations in genes. Despite all the advances in medical science over the years, the disappointing reality is that targeting mutations hasn't been the magic bullet it was thought to be, in part because the complex interaction between tumors and the microenvironment is still far from being fully understood. An oncologist colleague of mine recently said, "Lots of complex and complicated interactions occur at the tissue level that aren't yet completely understood; a deeper understanding of the biology is needed." While gene sequencing identifies mutations to aim at, it doesn't address the situation in which multiple mutations are present—a condition associated with disease progression and treatment response. (My colleague also echoed Dr. Ng's sentiment that a higher focus on the microbiome is needed).

Additionally, a group of noted luminaries in the field of oncology—the so-called Oncology Think Tank—believe a paradigm shift in the approach to cancer care is imperative and overdue, and so they are advocating for a radical change from the conventional, reactive approach (screening for select cancers in individual people) to a longitudinal, population-based one, across the spectrum of wellness to disease, wherein many cancers are detected early in their transition to malignancy, precancerous and/or early stages.

Considering that 40 percent of individuals eligible for CRC screening are not up to date, that viewpoint is understandable. One important consideration is that adopting a population-based strategy may involve endorsing a particular non-invasive test, which, while marginally less effective than other alternative options, could lead to increased screening participation. The balance between effectiveness, user-friendliness, and cost may be perceived differently when viewed from a population standpoint compared to an individual one.

Like normal, healthy cells, cancer cells want to live forever and their characteristic genomic and adaptive diversity gives them an evolutionary advantage that in some cancers can make a cure nearly impossible to develop. Recently, a clinician/researcher said to me that even the centuries old descriptive term "cancer" isn't really meaningful anymore, as each expression of the disease represents a different syndrome.

Despite the recent emergence and promise of better diagnostic tools and treatments, science is far from figuring out the "how" of cancer. The sobering fact is that only 15 percent of cancers have a clear genetic cause, while 85 percent are random alterations. Still, science is good at asking the "how" questions.

The "why" is perhaps a spiritual question.

# 23

# Two Suitcases

SHORTLY AFTER ASSUMING my physician executive role at St. Luke's in Boise in November 2015, I met another senior executive there, a man about my age. He was intelligent, had a quick grasp of complex issues, and flashed a lively sense of humor. But he could be curt and didn't suffer fools gladly. And he often seemed guarded. He had a shadowed corner that he didn't let new or casual acquaintances see into. Still, I liked him, and I felt that the feeling was mutual. The more we got to know each other, I sensed that just under his outward demeanor, there was sorrow and anger, perhaps even rage. As I eventually learned from a colleague, he had lost a son in his twenties to lymphatic cancer a few years before. At the time I learned this, the loss of a child seemed foreign (and almost incomprehensible) to me. Aside from "So sorry to hear that you lost a son," I didn't know what to say.

Population statistics show that by age 60, 9 percent of Americans have lost a child. Unlike the much more common shared experience of losing elderly parents, much of the road forward after such an event is a solo journey for the parents. You become part of a club that no one wants to join, aptly described elsewhere as the land of misfit parents.

A couple of times in the months after Patrick died, I had fleeting thoughts of killing myself to be reunited with him. I never formulated a plan. And I sometimes thought that if I knew that I would lose a child, I never would have become a parent. Today, I feel remorse about having had those horrific thoughts.

But as with the work colleague who had lost a son, I suppose I've been permanently concussed. I now have a range of simmering emotions about Patrick that can be triggered by an event, a word, a photograph, a song, unexpected memories—all spawning in turn anger, melancholy, fear and anxiety. Real tranquility only comes when I'm holding or observing my young grandchildren. A close friend of Kathy called them "mighty little healers."

My favorite pictures include one of my paternal grandfather, my adoptive father, me and Dan, then an infant—four generations spanning more than 70 years. I thought of that image often during a two-week vacation in August 2022 in an oceanfront rental in Chatham. The back of the house had a yard that sloped down to a shrubbery-lined border. A sandy path led to a private beach.

While sitting in a chair at the top of the slope, I had a great view of the yard, the beach, Pleasant Bay and the distant horizon. Watching Noah running on the beach and wading into the water with Charlie Flood provoked mixed emotions—I knew that Patrick should have been there—but overall, the sight of my living children on the beach with their children brought me great joy.

RESERVATIONS FOR NINE

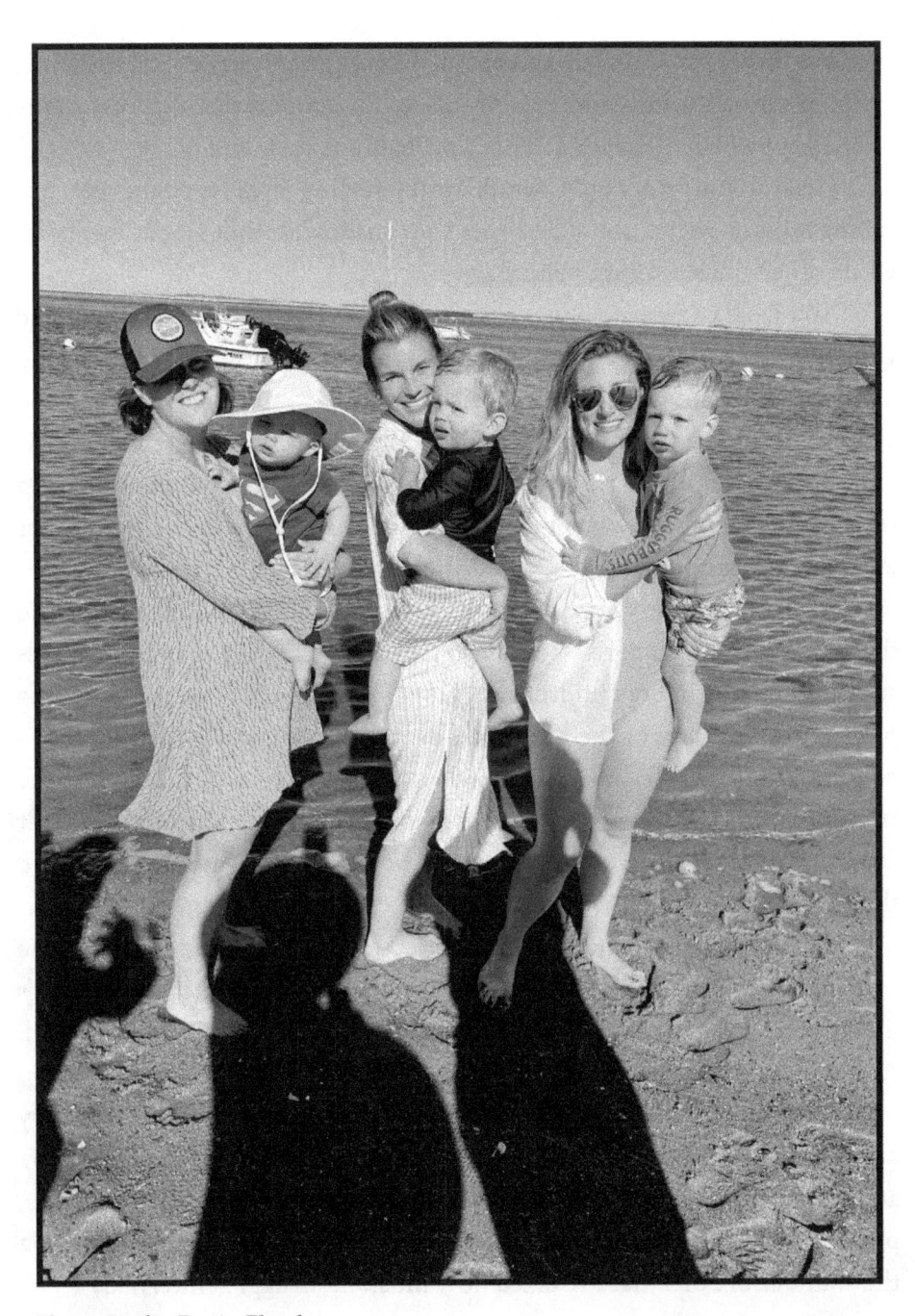

Photo Credit: Devin Flood

I've learned, and perhaps accepted, that my grief is irrepressible. While joyful experiences and moments of solace can temporarily suppress it, the grief can't be buried for long. That's probably as it should be.

Grief is fundamentally paradoxical—feeling it causes pain, yet, not feeling it hurts even more. It becomes your shadow; at times looming ahead, while other times trailing behind.

You have to figure out a way to move forward and help yourself and your family find a new equilibrium. That means reweaving your life into a cohesive and coherent pattern of hope-suffused emotions, thoughts and actions. You have to find a way to fill up the after as richly as the before.

Because Patrick's life started within Kathy's body and was born as a result of her labor, I knew her grief would be different from mine, perhaps even more tortuous in some ways. She envisions her future as a journey carrying two suitcases: one filled with joyful and cherished memories and the other laden with sorrow and loss. She talks of packing her happiness suitcase with joy in her children and grandchildren and consciously taking pleasure in so many of the quotidian events we often take for granted—conversations with friends, a delicious meal, a gorgeous day. Like me, she struggles with her faith, but she thinks our experience has increased her capacity for empathy. To her, love must be primary in the beginning and the end: it's about what we give to and receive from others.

Her grief suitcase, heavy with sadness, includes a sense of guilt—the continuing mistaken worry that she somehow contributed to Patrick's disease by, for example, not being vigilant enough about foods she served. And it carries the hole that is death, the absence of love.

My going forward is always spurred by Patrick's example and by sensing what his wishes would have been if he had lived. I recall how he admirably composed himself, even after his diagnosis: steadfast, selfless, positive, disciplined and poised. (It was only when I read his journal during the summer of 2023 that I realized how much he struggled internally). The last thing that he would want was grief dictating how I would conduct myself in his absence.

Still, there's a scene from an episode of the FX series *The Old Man* that resonated with me. An ex-CIA agent describes to a new acquaintance what he did before he started a new mission. He instructs the acquaintance to write her name on a paper napkin and stuff it into a glass of water. Somewhat reluctantly she does. The napkin contorts as it slowly absorbs the water.

They then talk about whether there's reversibility of the act and what it would mean in daily life thereafter.

Water often serves as a symbol of memory and the subconscious. I knew then that the scene represented my sometimes-buried memories of experiences that would continue to influence my life. These memories evoke my sense of identity and of what it means to survive life's storms as I try to come to terms with my experiences and connect their lessons with the present and future.

That's what having cancer—and having one of your children with cancer—feels like, and more.

Although in the months after Patrick's passing, I found less meaning in my work, that has changed. In my capacity as a physician executive, I don't see patients, but instead deal with strategic initiatives to improve the health of populations. Steering my thinking in that direction has helped provide a much-needed distraction from my swimming in the churning waters of grief. Even though I could have retired, I took on a new physician executive role in Connecticut and deferred retirement to keep active intellectually.

Kathy and I worried about the impact of Patrick's death on his brothers and sister. But as a family we share a lot about our feelings, and Dan, Kaylin and Brendan have all moved forward, albeit each carrying a suitcase of grief.

"I want to see Pat again," Dan wrote recently. "So bad. I lost my best friend. I would tell him that he is loved; his family is cared for; his friends still love and honor him and we will never stop. I would love to embrace my brother like I did at Parris Island, after a lacrosse win at Thayer, after a monumental lift at the gym, in South Boston after he proposed to Amanda, after I heard his cancer spread to his lungs. I would love to embrace him again. One more time."

Kaylin acknowledges that she struggles to find ways to cope with Patrick's death. Recently she wrote: "It doesn't feel like I have much control over my coping. Often, I will be driving alone and suddenly I am brought to tears. Most of my "moments" happen when I am alone. I hesitate to reach out to my parents in these moments because I don't want to bring them down if they happen to be "getting through" that day. I reach out to my brother, Brendan, more and more. There are times that I've arrived at my parents' house, and I'll go upstairs and just cry in front of him. He'll hold my hand or put a hand on my back and doesn't have to say anything at all.

"Moments when we're with the whole family can go either way. Sometimes, Pat's presence is so strong and there is a sense of comfort that he is there with us in spirit. Other times, his absence feels so obvious. There is no in between. And there is no in between with my coping, either. I'm either crying the hardest I've ever cried before, alone, struggling to catch my breath. Or I'm going about my day and not feeling flooded with grief. On those days, I can sing along to a song on the radio, I can be productive at work, I can show up for my family."

Brendan admits that his coping is "just something that all of us will be processing for the rest of our lives. While I'm incredibly thankful and fortunate to have a great support system, I still have this scar of sadness and pain and anger inside me, and a phantom boulder on my back.

"Personally, I've pinned my conversation history with Pat to the top of my messages on my phone because I am, even after three years, still so used to texting or calling him every day.

"Though it still and will always hurt, I believe that I am more at peace with my brother's passing. Patrick Beauregard lived a life anyone should and could strive to live. We'll keep going because that's what our family does. There is always hope, and we choose to always believe in that hope."

For my 65th birthday, Kaylin gifted me a subscription to Storyworth, a service that collects a person's favorite stories and memories and preserves them in a bound book. Storyworth recipients get weekly questions via email to write about. At the end of a year, the recipient receives a bound memoir of their stories. One of the questions I received was: How would you describe your children individually in one word? After thinking about it for several minutes, I wrote:

> Patrick: Indomitable
> Dan: Genuine
> Kaylin: Spirit
> Brendan: Destined

Every year since Patrick's death, we have held a memorial Mass in Chatham, presided over by Father Michael. Being with the Floods and seeing the friends of Patrick and Amanda always comforts us. This third year was the first service since the installation of Patrick's headstone.

The families stay together for several days at a large rental home in Chatham. During the year 2023, on the night before the Mass, the group assembled around a large dining room table. The children had been put to bed, so it was just adults with snacks, wine, whiskey and tequila. The conversation eventually became all about what people were feeling about Patrick.

Amanda, who has been so steadfast, so brave and committed to honoring her husband's life, usually keeps things close to the vest. But that evening she spoke candidly about what the past three years have been like. Her descriptions captured what Kathy and I had felt as well, albeit as parents and not as a spouse.

She described year one as "shocking" and everything that followed was "a blur." Year two was noteworthy for recognizing that many people (not immediate family) had already forgotten days that had meaning in Pat's life. Year three is all about the finality of it. The headstone in place is the ultimate symbol.

The tears that flowed—interspersed with memories of joyful moments and laughter—was a group cathartic release.

Life after the loss of a child is like walking across a vast borderless field scattered with surface markers that trigger strong memories and emotions. One can try to suppress such markers of time as birthdays, wedding anniversaries, and family holiday events. Yet, beneath the surface lie innumerable land mines, which can set off emotions that can derail an entire day, sending us into deep sorrow, and leaving us feeling overwhelmed. Coping with the many emotional ambushes are tough. One can try living strategically to avoid or suppress the aforementioned markers of time, but that's not exactly easy to pull off. Jocelyn, the psychologist who treated Kathy and me after my bladder cancer, taught us a valuable technique: We should take a moment to process our feelings before returning to the demands of the present.

I continue to struggle to manage emotions evoked by certain triggers, conscious and subconscious. For many years, I had taken pride in being called a calm and steady person. For the most part, I still am, but I have become more emotional in response to certain stimuli. Still, I'm making slow, steady progress. I could only bear recently to listen to the Stick Figure song "Paradise" without tearing up. The song—a reflection on life and a search for peace and happiness—is a favorite of my children. All I have is today, for which I'm grateful. I feel for the thousands of people who still have little hope because of the cancer that brought down Patrick and those with other lethal diseases.

During a recent trip to Europe, Kathy and I met many couples, and inevitably they asked if we had children. At first, the question always seemed to hang above us, as if suspended by a current of air, waiting to rise or fall depending on the response.

To avoid an unsettling silence, we needed, of course, to reply. It has taken time to fashion a reply that's adequate for the moment while holding our emotions in check: "We have had four children. Our oldest is 37. But we lost our second son at age 32 to colorectal cancer."

I remembered other advice from Jocelyn. You can't protect people from bad news; let them handle it themselves. Our honest response to friendly inquiries would quickly darken the faces of listeners as they struggled to respond in a meaningful way. However, in every instance, after a brief awkwardness, we moved the conversation to something light, such as the latest adventures of Dan, Kaylin and Brendan and—consistent with how grandparents most happily identify themselves—our grandchildren.

As our week in Europe continued, I was better able to utter the painful words about our loss of Patrick without my eyes welling up. We'll be asked well-intentioned questions about our family again, but I think we'll be ready to respond calmly and gracefully and often ask about questioners' families, too. I guess that's progress.

We try to have nuclear family dinners at our home once a month on a Sunday. During one in November 2022, and after other guests arrived, Amanda and Noah (then a little over two) arrived in the early afternoon. The day was cool, so Noah was wearing a sweatshirt. After he played with toys and ran around for a few minutes, Kathy noticed that he was sweating, so she helped him remove his sweatshirt. The words on his shirt underneath read, "Big Brother." After a few seconds of silence, people realized what that meant, gasped, and started cheering. Unbeknownst to us, Amanda, still committed to the desire she and Patrick shared to have three children, had gone through another IVF process and was pregnant! Noah would have a little brother.

On May 17, 2023, at 1:32 a.m. at Massachusetts General Hospital, after about a 22-hour labor, Colin Henry Beauregard came into the world weighing 7 pounds, 9 ounces. Roz and Kathy were in the room. The obstetrician asked Amanda who she wanted to cut the umbilical cord. Amanda and her mother said "Gma," the name Kathy wanted her grandchildren to call her. Kathy cut the cord, for Patrick.

Like his brother and his cousins as they grow up, Colin will know.

*In Loving Memory of Patrick Henry Beauregard*
*Born February 9th, 1988, in Portland, Maine*
*Died September 6th, 2020, in Medfield, Massachusetts*

# 24

# Afterword

DESPITE THE SIX-YEAR ordeal that began with seemingly innocuous abdominal pain in a healthy 29-year-old and culminated in tragedy, our family's story continues.

It has been four years since my son's heart ceased its timeless rhythm, succumbing to the relentless progression of a disease that began as a single abnormal cell in his mid teens. and stealthily progressed, insatiably, malevolently, and cruelly, into a disease that overwhelmed him.

I'd like to believe that, in the end, it wasn't cancer that took Patrick, but exhaustion from the relentless courage, determination and strength he poured into every moment of his three-year fight.

After the loss of a child, parents descend into a deep chasm of grief. One in which nearly each breath feels like a betrayal to their child's memory. Inescapable sorrow claws at their hearts and tears at their souls. The trust and belief in the goodness of the world are shattered, leaving a void filled with seemingly endless despair. Coping with the loss and attempting to mend the gaping wound left by the child's absence turns into an enormous challenge. Routine tasks seem insurmountable under the unyielding weight of grief.

There are times when it feels as if a void occupies the place where Patrick once stood—an emotional black hole whose gravitational pull tugs at the fragile fabric of our existence, consuming cherished memories and stealing future moments. Yet, his indomitable spirit remains, delicately woven into our family's foundation offering subtle strength and guiding us forward. In those moments, his presence provides the resilience to rest and recharge when it's most needed.

To label his passing as a defeat would be a disservice to his memory. Although the grief continues, as the years without him pass, I've perhaps gained a better acceptance that the way he dealt with his disease was his ultimate achievement.

But that doesn't stop me from repeating a phrase often spoken aloud by Kathy: *"It's so wrong. Why am I the one who's still here?"*

For Kathy and me, our sense of time has become diffuse. Kathy used to recall dates of important family events with remarkable accuracy, however long ago they were. I wasn't quite as precise, but I could still remember them fairly well. But now, time can seem distorted, and memories fragmented, with even our self-images sometimes recalling reflections in a funhouse mirror. Has it really been seven years since that fateful day in September 2017 when I heard the most terrifying sentence I'd yet heard? Have we really not seen our son for four years?

The reality of the phenomenon that claimed his life continues.

Across all races and ethnicities, trends in five-year relative survival rates for colorectal cancer in the U. S. in 1975–2019 improved to 64 percent from 50, most likely due to increased screening rates, which lead to diagnosis at lower stages which are more responsive to therapies.

A recent publication by the ACS showed that through 2021, overall cancer mortality has continued to decline. But the gains are imperiled by an increasing incidence of several of the leading cancer types. The incidence of colorectal cancers in adults under 50 continues to rise annually by 1–2 percent.

Age remains the strongest determinant of cancer risk. During 2019–2020, between age groups 65 and older, and 50 to 64, and younger than 50, only the under 50 group realized an increase in the overall incidence of cancer. In that same period, a 79 percent increase in the global incidence of early-onset cancer was observed. Accompanying that was a near 28 percent increase in early-onset cancer deaths.

A recent study shows that younger generations (so-called "birth cohorts" such as Millennials and Generation Xers) have seen larger increases in certain prime cancers compared to previous generations, suggesting high incidence rates may persist for decades, which begs the question: what changes in environmental substances and/or new epigenetic or immune system susceptibilities have emerged since the 1990s? The researchers stressed that they are still without a definitive explanation for the trend.

For colorectal cancer, the statistics remain grim. Since the late 90s, colorectal cancer has risen from being the fourth-leading cause of cancer death in men younger than 50 to being the first. In women younger than 50, it now trails only breast cancer. Its' rise to supplanting that as the lead cancer in women under 50 within a few years is a well justified concern. Perhaps, it's inevitable.

In 2024, for both sexes, estimates for new cases and deaths in people under 50 are 153,000 and 53,000 respectively. There are, however, no estimates of how many families and friends will be drawn into the maelstrom those cases incite. It evokes the medical term "too numerous to count".

Tireless research and development efforts are ongoing—and possessing a higher degree of urgency.

Since its inception in 2019, the DFCI Young-Onset Colorectal Cancer Center has evaluated about 1,400 patients. Grimly, the year-over-year numbers of new cases have been steadily rising, with the number in 2023 being 73 percent higher than in 2019. Astonishingly, some of the cases they've treated have been people under 20 years old. (Researchers have deemed it questionable that a colonic tumor could start developing in individuals aged 10–15 without a germline predisposition. Consequently, one hypothesis is that the interplay of the current exposome with an as-yet-undetermined set of individual risk factors during early life stages might trigger significant dysregulatory events, ultimately accelerating the onset of cancer during adolescence).

Dr. Ng recently shared with me that one reason she chose to specialize in adult oncology was her belief that treating children with cancer would be too emotionally challenging. Despite this decision, she now faces the difficult reality of treating an increasing number of patients who are under 20 years old.

Historically, financing for colorectal cancer research, both by governmental sources and public philanthropy has been underfunded. This issue remains particularly problematic. It's felt that this disease has been stigmatized. Plainly said, people don't like talking about intestines, rectums, and stool tests.

The 2023 Pan-Mass Challenge realized a record-breaking $72 million in donations—its largest gift ever—to the DFCI.

Meanwhile, the work of the Patrick Beauregard Foundation continues. In support of the PMC, riders of Team Panda Power raised nearly $57 thousand for the foundation. On Feb. 1, 2024, I proudly stood with a group of riders in a conference room in the Charles A. Dana building, on the grounds of the Yawkey Center for Cancer Care, in Boston, and watched Amanda present a check in that amount to Dr. Ng.

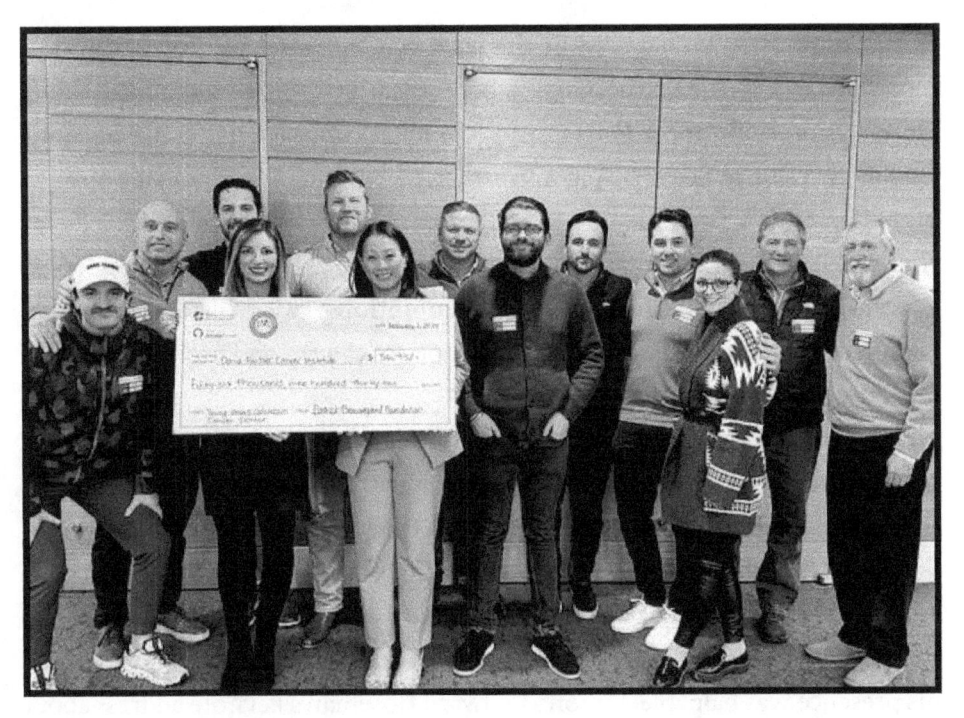

Courtesy: Dana-Farber Cancer Institute

A recent study identified four signs that were more commonly reported in people who were later diagnosed with colorectal cancer—abdominal pain, rectal bleeding, diarrhea and iron deficiency anemia. The presence of just one sign increased the risk two-fold; having all four signs resulted in a six-fold increase. In the 5,075 people who developed early-onset cancer, nearly 20 percent had one or more of the signs. (A similar analysis of adults aged 50–64 did not reveal the same association). Importantly, people with just one sign realized a (median) delay in diagnosis of nearly 10 months. Each additional sign shortened the time to diagnosis.

Of the stronger association in younger adults, Dr. Yin Cao, the study's senior investigator, said: [the findings suggest that among this population] "there's an avenue for early detection". She added that the findings underscore the importance of recognizing warning signs early.

## GEORGE BEAUREGARD

March 1, 2024, ushered in the start of Colorectal Cancer Awareness month. March 2, 2024, saw Dana Farber Cancer Institute's fifth annual Young Onset Colorectal Cancer Patient and Family Forum take place at The Hotel Commonwealth, in Boston. (A month earlier, the institute announced the opening of its Centers for Early Detection and Interception—a new, multidisciplinary clinical and research program that evaluates people at increased risk of developing cancer. Risks include previous genetic conditions, prior history of cancer, precursor conditions to cancer, family history of cancer, and positive results of a multi-cancer early detection test).

With burdened hearts, Kathy, Brendan, Amanda, and I attended, undeterred in our commitment to honor Patrick's legacy and to support the center's work for people stricken with this disease, their caregivers and families. I have become more adept at coping with the pain that comes with viewing the title slide of the welcome and opening remarks section of the forum, which depicts Patrick undergoing an examination by Dr. Ng. For me, his presence was palpable. Simone Ledward Boseman's keynote address about her experience as a caregiver for her deceased actor husband, Chadwick, who succumbed at age 43 from CRC, was brave, emotionally honest and inspiring, as were other stories told by other young adults affected by this cruel disease. I met two people who are five-year survivors and rejoiced for them.

April saw an interesting announcement of a prospective study that showed an association between accelerated aging, in which biological age (as determined by an algorithm utilizing 9 biomarkers found in blood) surpasses chronological age, and the rising incidence of early-onset cancers among people born during and after 1965. People with accelerated aging perhaps have an increased risk of developing early-onset cancer. If proven, interventions to brake biological aging could be a new path to cancer prevention.

Brendan will be in the field of runners participating in the 2024 Boston Marathon, this time as part of the DFCI team. He exceeded his initial fundraising goal of 15 thousand dollars by mid-February.

Although evidence-based effective screening methods for standard-onset CRC currently exist, the possibility of accelerated development of early-onset CRC raises pragmatic clinical considerations. Current screening protocols can only be effective for early-onset CRC if it develops along the classical adenoma-carcinoma cascade timelines.

Some promising novel approaches and techniques are under development: advanced technologies that improve the genetic analysis of stool samples, which may reveal the presence of tumor DNA, examining changes in the gut microbiome and identifying specific bacteria that might play a causative role in the cancer's development, and so-called liquid biopsies, tests that can detect, analyze, and track DNA and other substances shed from tumors into blood and urine. If proven successful, these non-invasive tests might also be used to assess treatment responses and resistance, as well as in post-treatment surveillance. The potential for more frequent testing with the possibility of performing a colonoscopy as a follow up procedure might be most relevant. In this regard, liquid biopsy monitoring might be effective for early detection of early-onset CRC.

In 2021, the Centers for Medicare and Medicaid (CMS) concluded that there was sufficient evidence to support the coverage of a blood-based biomarker test as a suitable CRC screening option for asymptomatic individuals at average risk. This test may be administered once every 3 years, provided it is conducted in a laboratory certified under the Clinical Laboratory Improvement Act (CLIA). Additionally, the test must be FDA approved and demonstrate both a true positive rate (sensitivity) of at least 74 percent and a true negative rate (specificity) of at least 90 percent for CRC.

Recently, following an FDA advisory committee's strong recommendation that the federal health agency approve Guardant Health's Shield blood test for early detection of colon cancer, the agency approved the test. Clinical trial data had demonstrated that the test had an 83 percent sensitivity rate; its specificity rate was just below 90 percent. A blood-based viable screening option now exists, particularly for people reluctant to have a colonoscopy or do a stool-based test.

While the FDA's decision will likely lead to higher rates of screening for colorectal cancer—and hopefully earlier detection of lower stages—, it presents several important issues that the physicians who will be ordering them will need to address. They will be seeking higher specificity and sensitivity along with substantial evidence that these innovative diagnostic tools significantly reduce the absolute incidence of higher-stage cancer with long-term, sustained benefits, ensuring no later-year cancer recurrence. All the while causing no harm to otherwise healthy people.

Another key consideration to early detection remains. To what extent will finding abnormal methylation—signaling a cancer formation or progression—be actionable? Can the cancer its heralding be located, reversed or eliminated? How useful are predictions that lack impactable interventions?

Although their potential is captivating, whether or not MCED tests will change the course of cancer screening, prevention and treatment remains to be seen.

For those under 45–a group in which screening is not recommended—a higher awareness of this burgeoning phenomenon is needed,

In the end, addressing the combined influences and interactions of concurrent exposures, genetic predispositions, and the fundamental processes of tumor development and evolutionary patterns in early-onset cancers presents a significant challenge.

The Beauregard family continues to move forward, making new strides and memories while preserving the past. A memorial ceremony for Patrick occurs every first week in September in Chatham with Father Michael saying Mass.

Patrick's framed photograph sits on the tabletop at every family gathering meal.

# 25

# Acknowledgments

ALONG THE WAY of this labor of love and grief, I have been greatly helped by many people.

To my excellent editor, Richard Babcock. Dick, I understand what you meant when you said "God is in the rewrite".

Thank you to Robert Whitcomb, whose support, experience, sage wisdom, candor, advice, and friendship have been invaluable during this writing journey.

A special thank you to Mary Walsh, whose encouragement and support through multiple drafts, revisions, conversations, and angst kept me going during the times when the writing was really hard.

And last but not least, to all those whose vocation is health care. Despite the harsh realities and challenges that it brings at times, the sense of purpose and fulfillment that accompanies it is incomparable. There's no greater calling than caring for other people—the vast majority of which are complete strangers—in their time of need. Just saying thank you feels inadequate, but I know you're not in it for recognition and glory.

# 26

# Bibliography

THE BOOK NEVER would have been possible without having Patrick's own words to describe his ordeal. His public-facing journal divulged his experiences, thoughts and emotions and provided insight into how he and Amanda were dealing with his circumstances. His private journal entries went several layers deeper; they excavated and surfaced the root caps of his deepest emotions and mindsets throughout his ordeal.

Sources in the bibliography coincide with the chapter in which they appear in the book.

## All We Have Is Today

Siegel RL, Sandeep Wagle N, Cercek A, Smith RA, Jemal A. "Colorectal cancer statistics, 2023." *CA Cancer J Clin 2023; 1–22*

U.S. Preventive Services Task Force. Screening for colorectal cancer: US Preventive Services Task Force recommendation statement. *JAMA.* May 18, 2021. Volume 325, Number 19

Ugai T, Sasamoto N, Lee HY, Ando M, et al. "Is early-onset cancer an emerging global epidemic? Current evidence and future implications." *Nature Reviews* October 2022. Volume 19; 656–673

Erika Edwards. "As colon cancer spreads in younger adults, new research identifies earliest symptoms." *NBC News* article May 4, 2023

Mauri G, Patelli G, Sartore-Bianchi A. et al. "Early-onset cancers: Biological bases and clinical implications." *Cell Reports Medicine 5* September 17, 2024; 1–14

## Misbehaving Cells

Siegel RL, Miller KD, Fuchs HE, Jemal A. Cancer Statistics, 2021. *CA Cancer J Clin 2021 Jan;71(1):7–33*

## On Being a Doctor

Phillips, K, Ospina, N, Montori, V. "Physicians Interrupting Patients." *J Gen Int Med,* Oct 2019; 34 (10)

Groopman, J. (2007) "How Doctors Think." Houghton Miffin, 2007.

## Looking for a Breakthrough

Fagerberg B, et al. "Effect of metoprolol CR/XL in chronic heart failure: Metoprolol CR/XL Randomised Intervention Trial in Congestive Heart Failure". *The Lancet. 1999. 353(9169):2001–7.*

Rossouw JE, Anderson GL, Prentice RL, et al. Risks and benefits of estrogen plus progestin in healthy postmenopausal women: principal results From the Women's Health Initiative randomized controlled trial. *JAMA. 2002 Jul 17;288(3):321–33.*

Densen P. "Challenges and opportunities facing medical education." *Trans Am Clin Climatol Assoc. 2011; 122:48–58.*

## Frontiers of Hope

Kong C, Liang L, Liu G, Du L, et al. "Integrated metagenomic and metabolomic analysis reveals distinct gut-microbiome-derived phenotypes in early-onset colorectal cancer." *Gut 2023; 72: 1129–1142*

Zhao, LY, Mei, JX, Yu, G, et al. "Role of gut microbiota in anticancer therapy: from molecular mechanisms to clinical applications." *Signal Transduction and Targeted Therapy May 2023; Vol 8, 1–27*

Nicholson BD, Oke J, Virdee PS, Harris DA et al. "Multi-cancer early detection tests in symptomatic patients referred for cancer investigation in England and Wales (SYMPLIFY): a large-scale, observational cohort study." *Lancet Oncology Vol 24 July 2023: 733–743*

Klein EA, Richards D, Cohn A, et al. "Clinical validation of a targeted methylation-based multi-cancer early detection test using an independent validation set." *Ann Oncol. 2021 Sep;32(9):1167–1177*

Singhal, A., Li, B.T. & O'Reilly, E.M. Targeting KRAS in Cancer. *Nat Med 30, 969–983 (2024).*

Galsky MD, Daneshmand S, Izadmehr S, et al. "Gemcitabine and cisplatin plus nivolumab as organ-sparing treatment for muscle-invasive bladder cancer: a phase 2 trial." *Nat Med 29, 2825–2843 (2023)*

Ledford H. "Cancer trial results show power of weaponized antibodies." *Nature Vol 623, 231–232 (2023)*

Qaseem, A, Harrod, CS, Crandall, CJ, et al; "Clinical Guidelines Committee of the American College of Physicians. Screening for Colorectal Cancer in Asymptomatic Average-Risk Adults: A Guidance Statement From the American College of Physicians" *Ann Intern Med 2023;176:1092–1100*

Barot, SV, Sangwan, N, Nair, KG, et al. "Distinct intratumoral microbiome of young-onset and average-onset colorectal cancer." *Lancet eBioMedicine Feb 2024;100: 1–12*

Wu, WKK, Yu, J, "Microbiota-based biomarkers and therapeutics for cancer management." *Nat Rev Gastroenterol Hepatol 21, 72–73 (2024).*

Harris E. "Bacterial Subspecies Linked With Aggressive Colorectal Cancer Tumors." *JAMA. Published online April 19, 2024. doi:10.1001/jama.2024.5928*

Corcoran, RB, "A single inhibitor for all KRAS mutations." *Nat Cancer, 2023 Aug;4(8):1060–1062.*

Desai, J, Alonso, G, Kim, SH, et al. "Divarasib plus cetuximab in *KRAS G12C*-positive colorectal cancer: a phase I b trial." *Nat Med 30, 271–278 (2024)*

Chalabi, M, Verschoor, YL, van den Berg, J, et al. "LBA7 Neoadjuvant immune checkpoint inhibition in locally advanced MMR-deficient colon cancer: The NICHE- 2 study." *Ann Onc 2022. 08.16.*

"Turning the tide of early cancer detection." *Nat Med 30, 1217 (2024)*

## Afterword

Jensen TS, et al. Decision Memo for Screening for Colorectal Cancer—Blood-Based Biomarker Tests. CAG-00454N. January 19, 2021.

Fritz CDL, Otegbeye EE, Zong X, et al. "Red-flag signs and symptoms for earlier diagnosis of early-onset colorectal cancer." *J Natl Cancer Inst.* 2023 August 8;115(8):909–916

Siegel RL, Gianquinto AN, Jemal A. "Cancer statistics, 2024." *CA Cancer J Clin.* 2024; 1–38

Zhao J, Xu L, Sun J, et al. Global trends in incidence, death, burden and risk factors of early-onset cancer from 1990 to 2019. *BMJ Oncology* 2023;2:e000049.

Accelerated aging may increase the risk of early-onset cancers in younger generations. *American Association of Cancer Research News Release.* April 7, 2024

Sung, H., Siegel, R. L., Rosenberg, P. S., & Jemal, A. (2019). Differences in cancer rates among adults born between 1920 and 1990 in the USA: an analysis of population-based cancer registry data. *The Lancet Public Health*, 4(9), e495–e503.

Rosenberg PS, Miranda-Filho A. Cancer Incidence Trends in Successive Social Generations in the U.S. *JAMA Netw Open.* 2024;7(6):e2415731. do:10.1001/jamanetworkopen.2024.15731

Chung DC, Gray DM II, Singh H, et al. "A cell-free DNA blood-based test for colorectal cancer screening." *N Engl J Med 2024; 390:973–983*

*What is essential does not die but clarifies. The greatest tribute to the dead is not grief but gratitude."*

—*Thornton Wilder (1927)*

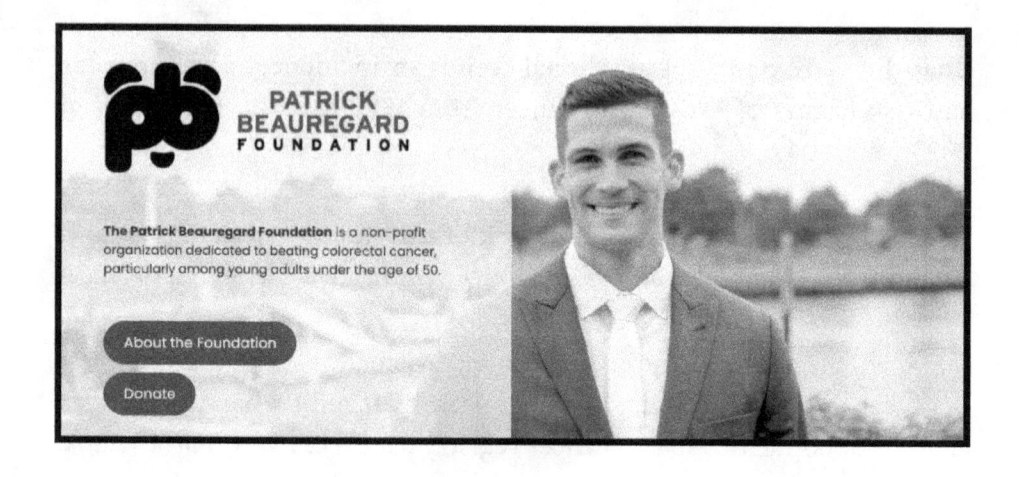

### PATRICK BEAUREGARD FOUNDATION

**The Patrick Beauregard Foundation** is a non-profit organization dedicated to beating colorectal cancer, particularly among young adults under the age of 50.

About the Foundation

Donate

# DEDICATIONS

*To Kathy, Daniel, Patrick, Kaylin and Brendan: Your presence has been and continues to be, the essence of my life. The real reason why I was born, and fought so hard to survive.*

*To Amanda, Melissa and Paul: Your additions to our family serve as priceless gifts that have enriched Kathy and my lives beyond what words can describe. Continue to take great care of the sons and daughter that we love so much.*

*For all my grandchildren: Noah, Camden, Miles, Isabelle, and Colin. Truly our "mighty little healers". You will all know.*

*In fond memory of Rodolphe (Rudy) and Marguerite (Peg) Beauregard: It's impossible to imagine what my life would've been like without you. I draw comfort and solace from my belief that you have been present and providing love and support for all of us from your place in heaven.*

*For Gary, my brother of 31 years: if only you had lived long enough to the time when HIV became just another chronic illness rather than a death sentence. Your work did not go unnoticed.*

GEORGE BEAUREGARD

*For the Flood family: Your collective love and support has been a treasure. What we have endured together during the past several years binds us forever.*

*For all the members of Team Panda Power: Never forget the words of your Captain: "Never give up."*

*To Kimmie Ng, MD and all the researchers and clinical and support staff at Dana-Farber. We are eternally grateful for the superb care you provided to our son and all of the other patients who come through your door. There's no doubt in my mind that your legacy will include finding the cause and cure of this disease.*

*To Mother Olga of the Sacred Heart, the Sisters of Mary of Nazareth and Father Michael Zimmerman: Your presence, love, support and profound healing influence on our lives defies description. You are all a permanent and treasured part of our family.*

*For John K. Erban III, MD: a dear friend, a colleague and my savior. Also taken too soon at age 65 by cancer. Hope you are resting in peace.*

*And last but not least: For those afflicted by early onset colorectal cancer: I'm so sorry that you have to bear this undeserved burden. But do not let cancer control you. As Patrick said: "If you're a patient, a survivor or caregiver…if you're still out there fighting…, know that you're not alone, so keep fighting and never give up."*

# TESTIMONIAL

## Congressional Record
## House of Representatives

Tuesday, Sept. 15, 2020

Massachusetts Congressman James P. McGovern

*Mr. Speaker, I rise today with a heavy heart to honor the life and service of a truly exceptional young man whom I had the great fortune of meeting and working with, Patrick Henry Beauregard, who was taken from us far too soon on September 6, 2020 after a courageous and awe-inspiring battle with colorectal cancer. Many of you know that my own faith has been greatly influenced by the teachings of the Jesuits, and in particular the idea that we ought to live our lives as "Men and Women for others." Mr. Speaker, Patrick Beauregard embodied this idea in every way.*

*Patrick was born in Portland, Maine and grew up in Medfield, Massachusetts. He attended Thayer Academy in Braintree, Massachusetts and Providence College in Providence, Rhode Island, where he met the love of his life Amanda. After graduating from college, Patrick decided to serve our country by enlisting in the United States Marine Corps, where he was an intelligence analyst. During his* service, Patrick received commendations for exceptional leadership, initiative, loyalty, and dedication to duty.

Patrick's Stage IV Colorectal Cancer diagnosis in September 2017 at the age of 29, a month after marrying his beloved wife Amanda, changed everything. I think so many of us would be tempted to give in to the uncertainty and doubt, but Patrick Beauregard remained positive through surgeries, immunotherapy and over 40 rounds of chemotherapy.

But what inspires me most about Patrick is that in the midst of this awful situation, he saw an opportunity to do good. Even as he fought his own disease with incredible grace and resilience, he used his voice to speak out, and to bring the issue of colorectal cancer to the attention of researchers, donors, elected officials, and other young people at risk for this disease. He appeared on the news, advocated for patients, and worked with groups like the Prevent Cancer Foundation to educate the public about the alarming increase of young onset Colorectal Cancer.

Mr. Speaker, Patrick Beauregard truly lived his life in service to others. From serving on the Alumni Association Board at Thayer Academy, to serving in the United States Marine Corps, to serving as an advocate so that we can prevent this terrible disease, Patrick is an inspiration to all of us, and he embodies the ideas of service and self-sacrifice this nation was built on. His incredible strength and tenacity allowed him to accomplish his final goal of meeting his son, Noah Patrick, on July 10, 2020. Noah—your dad was a great man , but more importantly, he was a very good man who did his very best to serve those around him and made our world a better place.

On behalf of the people of Massachusetts, cancer patients and survivors around the world, and the entire United States Congress, please join me in honoring the life and service of Patrick Henry Beauregard and praying for his family, friends, and all those who hold him in their heart."

# PRAISE FOR RESERVATIONS FOR NINE

"Dr. George Beauregard has penned a book in blood, sweat and tears. His stirring account of his son Patrick's extraordinary life and fierce battle with cancer incorporates his own expertise as a doctor and his own experience as a cancer survivor. The emperor of all maladies, cancer colonizes its victims and upends family and social life. In this poignant and life-affirming chronicle, Dr. Beauregard gives cancer patients and their families a compass and a map to make their way through the wilderness of cancer and its treatment. This is a true labor of love."

**—Congressman Jamie Raskin (MD-08),**
**author of** *Unthinkable: Trauma, Truth and the Trials*
*of American Democracy,* **New York Times #1 Bestseller.**

"Reservations for Nine" is a heartfelt story about a family's enduring love in the face of cancer. This book centers around Patrick, who, at age 29, is diagnosed with stage 4 colorectal cancer. Patrick's father—the author, is a physician and a cancer survivor himself. He uses his knowledge and experience to support his son through navigating the healthcare system, numerous rounds of chemotherapy, clinical trials, all of the time deeply appreciating the joy of being a father and the importance of faith and love on the journey.

The battle does not end with Patrick's passing, his father continues the fight to increase awareness about young-onset colorectal cancer screening, assessment, and effective treatment. He harnesses the energy generated from this very painful journey to motivate himself and others to raise awareness, promote funding for research, and offer compassionate support to those affected by this disease. As Margaret Mead has shared "Never Doubt That a Small Group of Thoughtful, Committed Citizens Can Change the World; Indeed, It's the Only Thing That Ever Has." Dr Beauregard is leading this charge, and important changes are occurring as a result of his efforts.

The book is a testament to the enduring power of love, compassion, and the importance of using hard experiences to improve the lives of many others. Patrick's legacy, intertwined with his father and family's unwavering dedication, serves as a powerful reminder that even amidst profound loss, hope and purpose can emerge. Those experiencing cancer and the journey it requires and those who are inspired by the love and compassion family and faith can make are highly encouraged to read this book."

**—Scott Conard, MD, Professor Emeritus UT Southwestern Department of Community and Family Medicine**

"This is a poignant and very personal story about parents of a close-knit family losing a courageous son to colorectal cancer all too soon. It is an important call to arms for all of us, including the medical establishment, for earlier, better and more accessible diagnostic testing to curtail the vast escalation in the young adult onset of this deadly disease. A highly impactful read."

**—Jeffrey Hogan, President, Upside Health Advisors**

"Cancer will soon overtake cardiovascular disease as the number one cause of death in the U.S. and the number of early-onset cancers among young people has exploded. The days of cancer being a disease of the elderly is gone; scientists are struggling with understanding the rise of cancers in otherwise healthy persons under age 50. Health systems across the nation, scientists and providers from all disciplines should be compelled to establish program-specific "young onset cancer" programs like the one Pat Beauregard helped launch at Dana-Farber Cancer Institute to address the alarming increases in cancer among children, teens and young adults.

Pat Beauregard was in the prime of his life, a United States Marine, healthy with no apparent risk factors, and one month after his wedding when he learned of his stage IV colon diagnosis. "Reservations for Nine", written poignantly by Pat's physician father, captures a family's heart-rending experience in dealing with their 29-year-old son's valiant three-year battle with cancer. Their collective journey as a family who pulled out all the stops in tackling Pat's disease is profoundly moving. As heart-stirring, is Pat's selfless mission over these three years to raise awareness for early detection and treatment.

Pat's diagnosis coincided with my sister-in-law's stage IV colon cancer diagnosis. Like Pat, she was healthy, age 45 with no family history or risk factors, a mother with young children. Her husband, also a physician, frequently compared notes with Pat's father on treatment strategies, both traditional and novel. Like the Beauregard family, my brother's family has been profoundly impacted by the sudden diagnosis and loss of their young wife and mother.

Dr. Beauregard's book is an inspiring and exquisite testament to his son and underscores Pat's mission in his final years to raise much-needed awareness and early detection of this early-onset cancer phenomenon. It also highlights the hope that Pat's legacy will help inform medical advances that change the way patients are screened and treated."

—**Rebecca Harrington, Co-Founder & President, The Leadership Institute**

"A harrowing story of a doctor and father and his son caught in the rising wave of young onset colon cancer. A must-read for any family confronting cancer in the prime of life."

—Dan Zuckerman, MD, FASCO, Director,
GI Oncology, St. Luke's Cancer Institute

"Reservations for Nine" is a deeply powerful narrative that profoundly blends medical insight with raw personal experience. George Beauregard's story of his family's battle with cancer is both heart-wrenching and inspiring. The book is testament to the resilience of the human spirit, the unbreakable strength of family, and the enduring power of hope. As a researcher dedicated to early-onset colorectal cancer prevention and risk factor discovery, I found this book exceptionally resonant. It calls on all of us to raise awareness and prioritize early detection, reminding us that cancer is no longer just a disease of the elderly. This fight is urgent, and we must act now."

—Yin Cao, ScD, MPH, Associate Professor of Surgery,
Division of Public Health Sciences,
Department of Surgery,
Washington University School of Medicine

"Having lost my mother to colorectal cancer, I understand the devastating impact it can have on the entire family. In this poignant and deeply moving account, Dr. Beauregard shares his uniquely personal perspective as a father and medical doctor grappling with his young son's colorectal cancer journey. Dr. Beauregard's eloquent storytelling is engaging, heart-wrenching and insightful. I applaud his courage in writing this book and creating greater awareness of the rising rates of colorectal cancer in younger adults. We all need to take action to end this disease."

—**Michael Sapienza**

"Movie-star handsome, charismatic newlywed Marine Pat Beauregard was blindsided at 29-years-old with advanced colorectal cancer, a disease mysteriously impacting young people at an alarming rate.

Pat selflessly spent time—his most precious asset—working with the medical community, the Prevent Cancer Foundation and the media to educate the public and inspire action. His story is continued here as his loving father—himself a physician—turns heartache into hope and underscores the need to prevent cancer and detect it early for better outcomes.

For me this book is deeply personal. Just a year after I began working with Pat to raise awareness about early-onset colorectal cancer, my own 18-year-old daughter was diagnosed with a rare cancer. Patrick became our North Star in navigating the vast, deep, dark waters. His father continues this legacy by making these diseases more understandable, using relatable analogies to explain complicated science.

This deeply touching book is a must-read for anyone dealing with a cancer diagnosis in their family, and an inspiring guide to advocating aggressively for the best possible care—as individuals and as a country."

—**Lisa McGovern, Executive Director,
Prevent Cancer's Congressional Families Program**

"With the rising incidence of early-onset colorectal cancer, George writes a comprehensive and personal story of not only the challenges of what our patients experience, but also the science of the emerging data on why this phenomenon is being observed. This is a must read for anybody treating young patients with cancer, and this book drives home the importance of compassionate care, incredible courage, and the inspiration our patients provide the world every single day."

—**Christopher Lieu, MD, Professor of Medicine,
GI Medical Oncology,
University of Colorado Cancer Center**

"My interview with Patrick always reminded me of my brother who died from colorectal cancer at 46. They both shared a spirit of tenacity, hope, and an undying will to live. George Beauregard's viewpoint as a physician, cancer survivor and father, provides unique insight into how this insidious disease impacts the patient, the family and friends. A must read."

—**Mark Ockerbloom, Anchor/Boston 25 News**

"The numbers and statistics behind the rise in young-onset colorectal cancer are frightening, but nothing quite hammers home the devastation that this disease brings to a young person and their family like this touching memoir of a father grappling with the diagnosis of metastatic colorectal cancer in his 29 year-old newlywed son, Pat. The story that lies within these pages poignantly describes the impact of young-onset colorectal cancer from many perspectives, including Pat himself, his young wife Amanda, his parents, and his siblings. The light that shines through it all, though, is the healing power of advocacy, which was infused throughout Pat's brave battle with young-onset colorectal cancer and is now infused throughout his father's book to raise awareness and advocate for scientific progress, prevention, and early detection."

—**Kimmie Ng, MD, MPH, Director, Young-Onset Colorectal Cancer Center & Director of Clinical and Biospecimen Research, Gastrointestinal Cancer Center at Dana-Farber Cancer Institute, Associate Professor of Medicine, Harvard Medical School**

"Cancer comes into millions of homes every year, and "Reservations for Nine" tells a poignant story of one family's long and arduous battle against the disease, marked by both heartbreak and resilience. There is no avoidance here—the story is raw and powerful. At the heart of this narrative is the son's steadfast and selfless dedication to advocating for greater awareness and funding for cancer research. Additionally, the book provides valuable insights into recognizing subtle cancer symptoms, empowering readers to seek the best possible treatment for themselves and their loved ones.

As a researcher, an oncologist, and a cancer widow, I am all too aware of the profound anguish cancer inflicts upon people and their families. The fact that it is now affecting younger people not only heightens the need for raising awareness, but more importantly, reaffirms the need for a new approach to cancer research be taken; one in which scientists focus their efforts on finding ways to detect and treat the earliest origins of cancer, rather than just devising treatments of established stage disease. Individuals, families, health-care providers, researchers, and policymakers would benefit from keeping this family saga close at hand. As James Bryce famously stated, "The worth of a book is to be measured by what you can carry away from it."

—Azra Raza MD
Chan Soon-Shiong Professor of Medicine
Clinical Director, Edward P. Evans Foundation MDS Center
Columbia University Medical Center
Author of "The First Cell: And the Human
Costs of Pursuing Cancer to the Last"

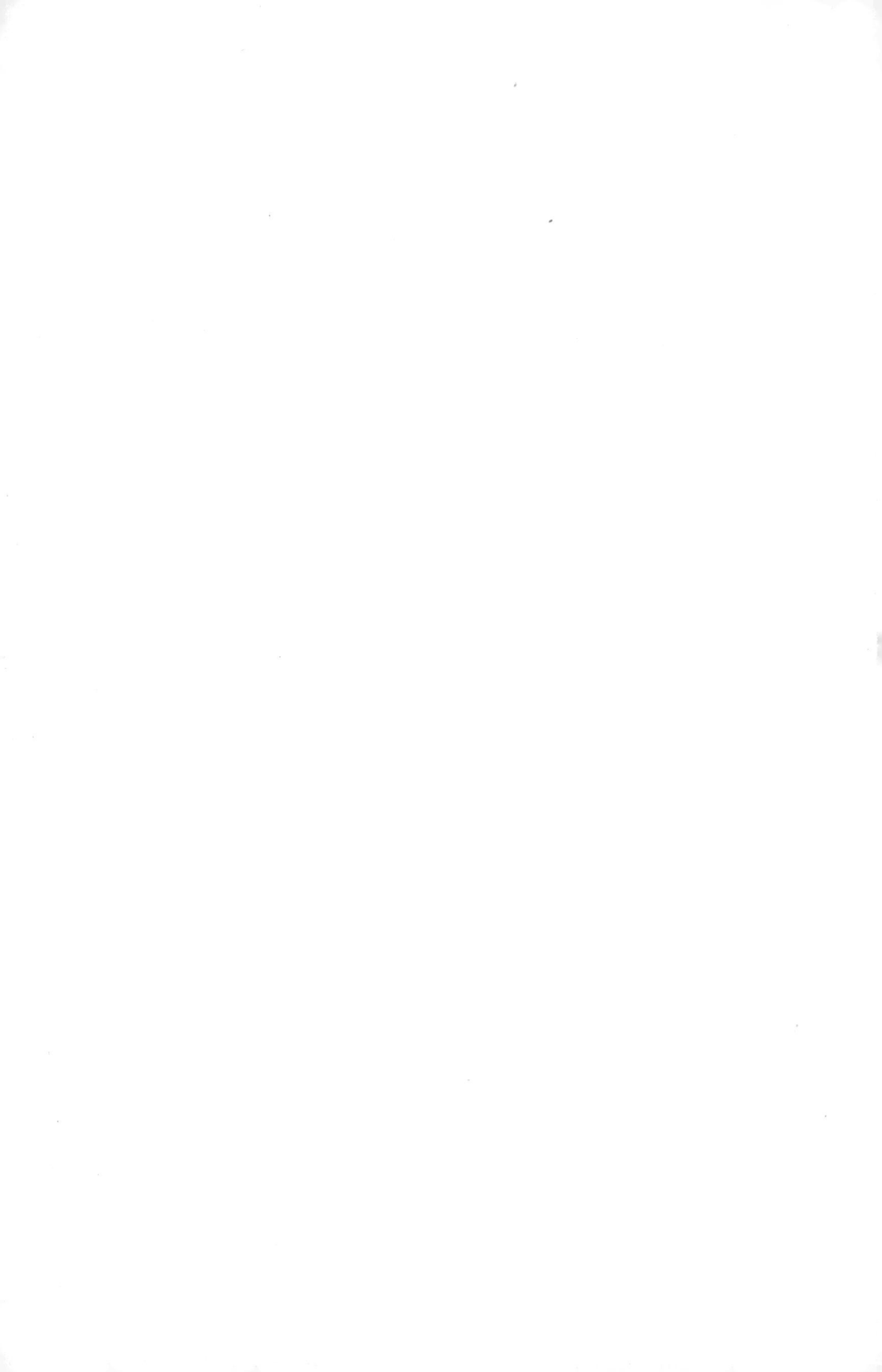